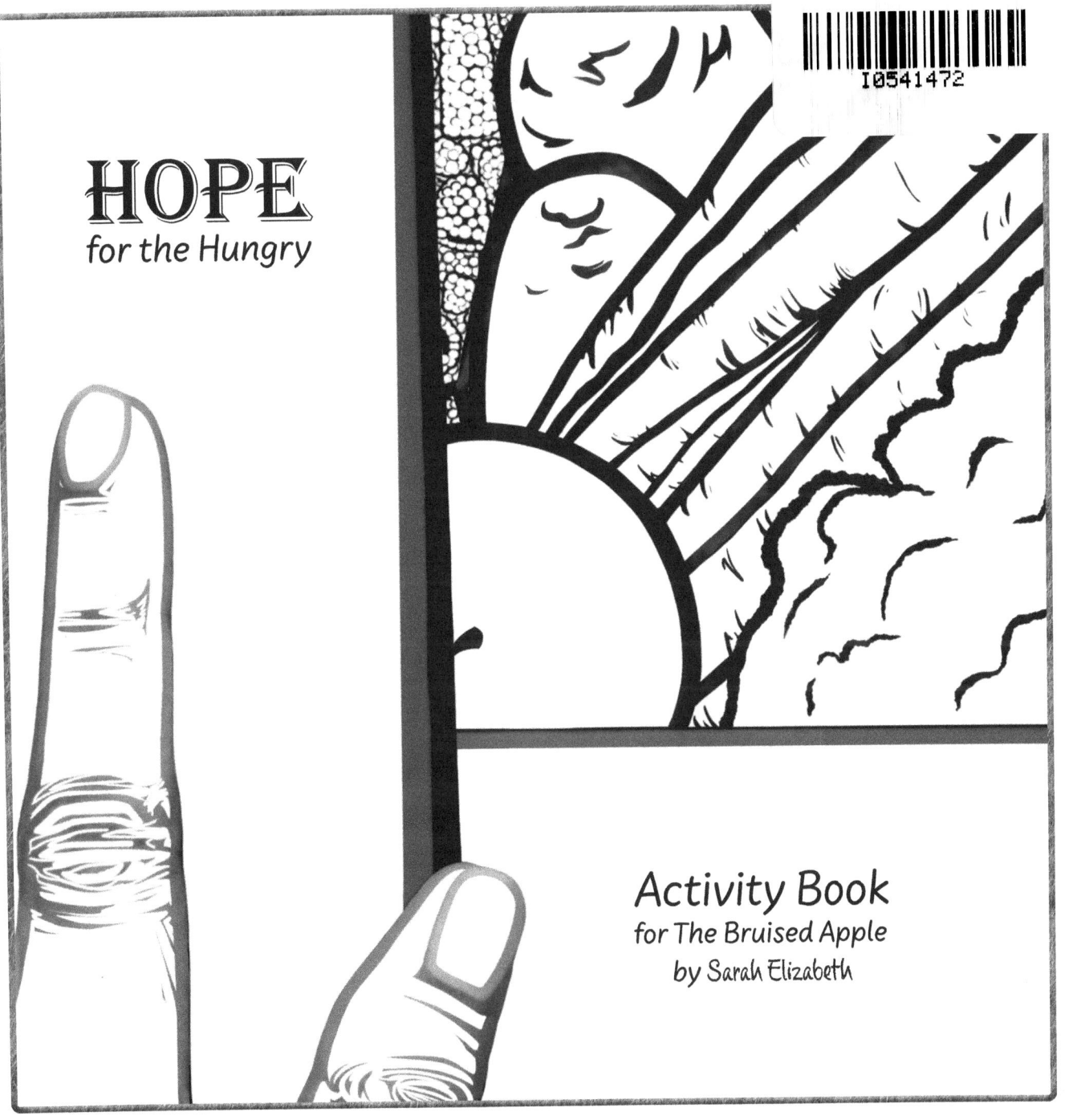

HOPE
for the Hungry

Activity Book
for *The Bruised Apple*
by Sarah Elizabeth

ISBN: 979-8-9854728-2-0

Published by Sarah Elizabeth
sarah.elizabeth@twinklingsofhope.com

To all who hunger for hope.

Hello, dear reader!

You're free to do however little or much you want of these activities and readings, but, especially when there seems to be too much, remember that each part is truly meant to help! Can you imagine how the following picture would turn out with just 60 dots? 40? 20? The fewer there are to connect, the more blockish it would look. Likewise, everything in this book helps share the message more fully and enhances its clarity. Another thing to note from the dot activity is that certain dots have the line return to them, like how 33 goes back through dot 29. Some things in this book will be repeated too, but it's always purposeful.

As to the point, this is to make known the hope of the mother in *The Bruised Apple*, hope that is not mere storybook hope since it is grounded in and grown from truth and trustworthy assurances. This activity book is meant to be worked through from beginning to end (but not in one sitting!!). It's important and even necessary for the middle section, at least, to be read before the last section. Thank you!

Parents and guardians, while I mean for this book to be helpful to you, it may not be the way you want to have your kid(s) be introduced to these matters. That may be the case even if you do believe the message is true and faithfully shared. What you do with it is, of course, up to you.

Thanks again! Take care.

Sincerely,

Sarah Elizabeth

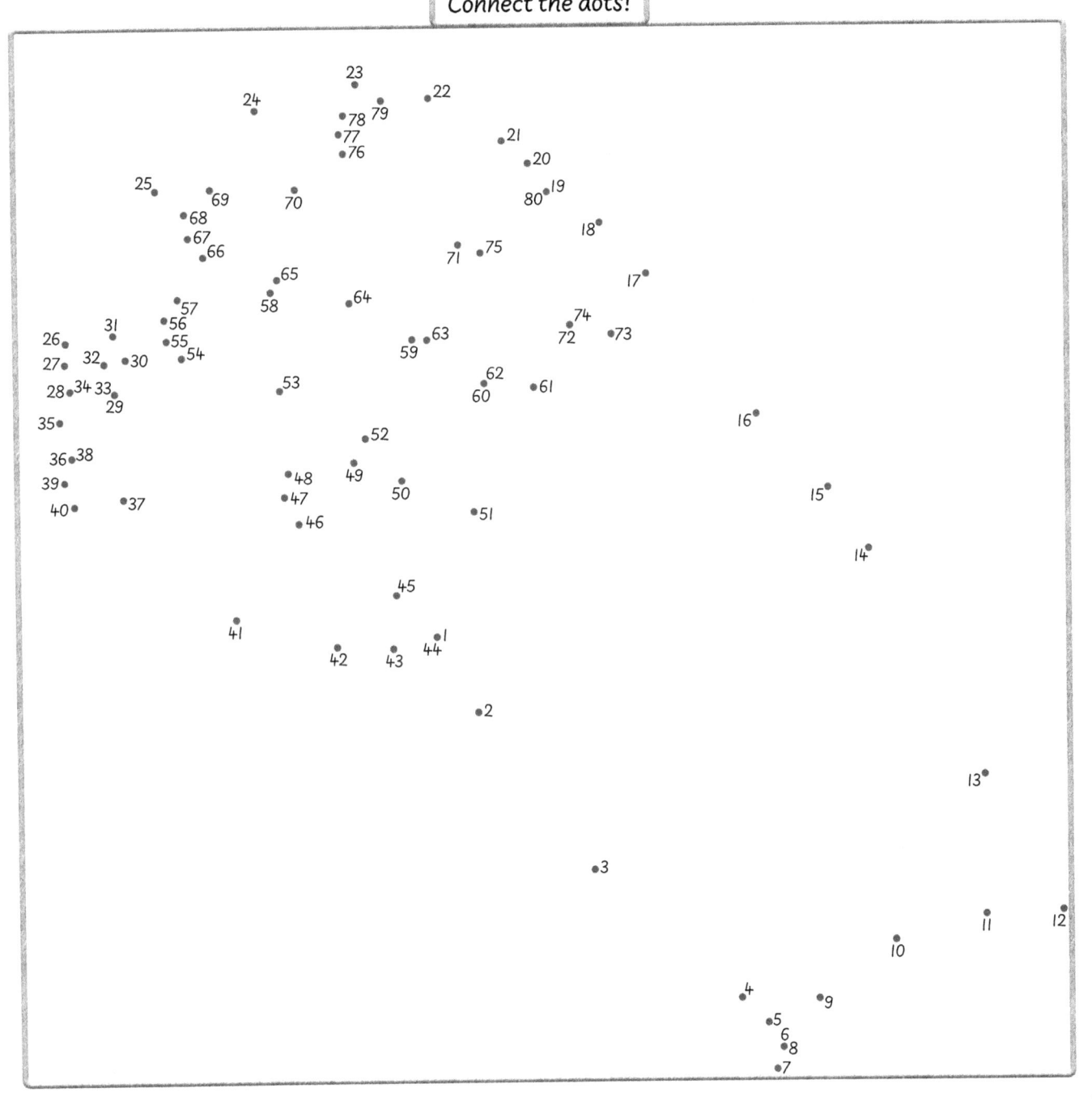

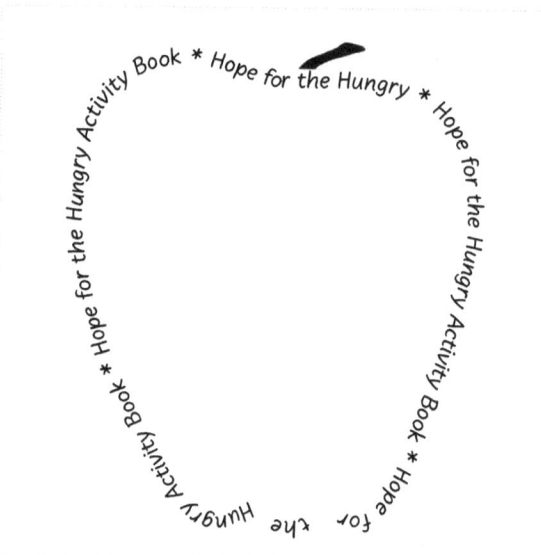

Hope for the Hungry Activity Book * Hope for the Hungry * Hope for the Hungry Activity Book * Hope for the Hungry Activity Book

Food Banks and Hunger

Tons of uneaten food gets trashed, but

food banks,

with the help of their partners,

rescue food that still could be eaten

from some stores,

restaurants,

and farmers.

Volunteers and workers sort it all

by standards to decide what they keep.

And, though not for people, what's tossed might

feed the soil instead of a trash heap.

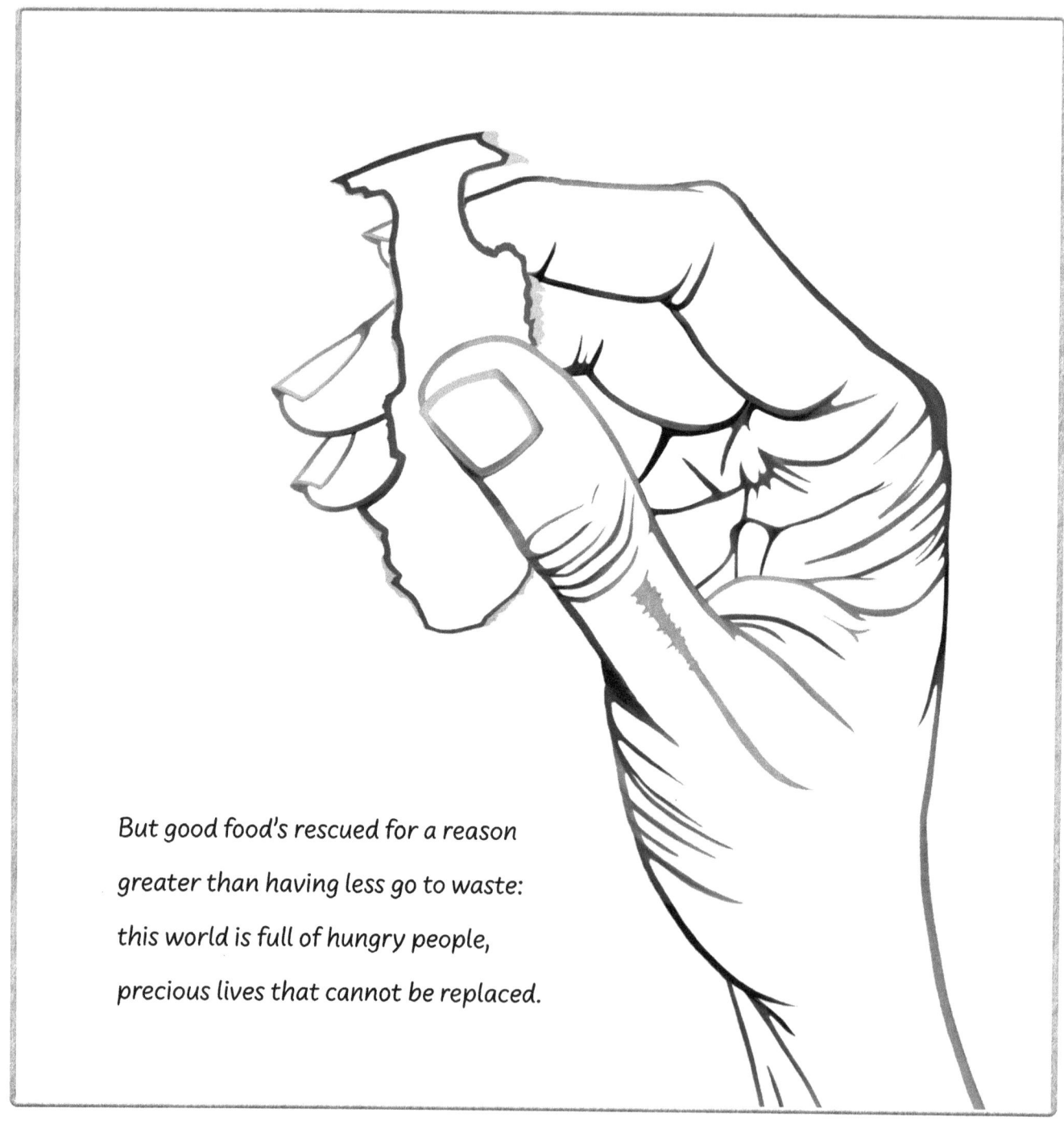

But good food's rescued for a reason
greater than having less go to waste:
this world is full of hungry people,
precious lives that cannot be replaced.

Circle or color what you think a food bank might want from these items.

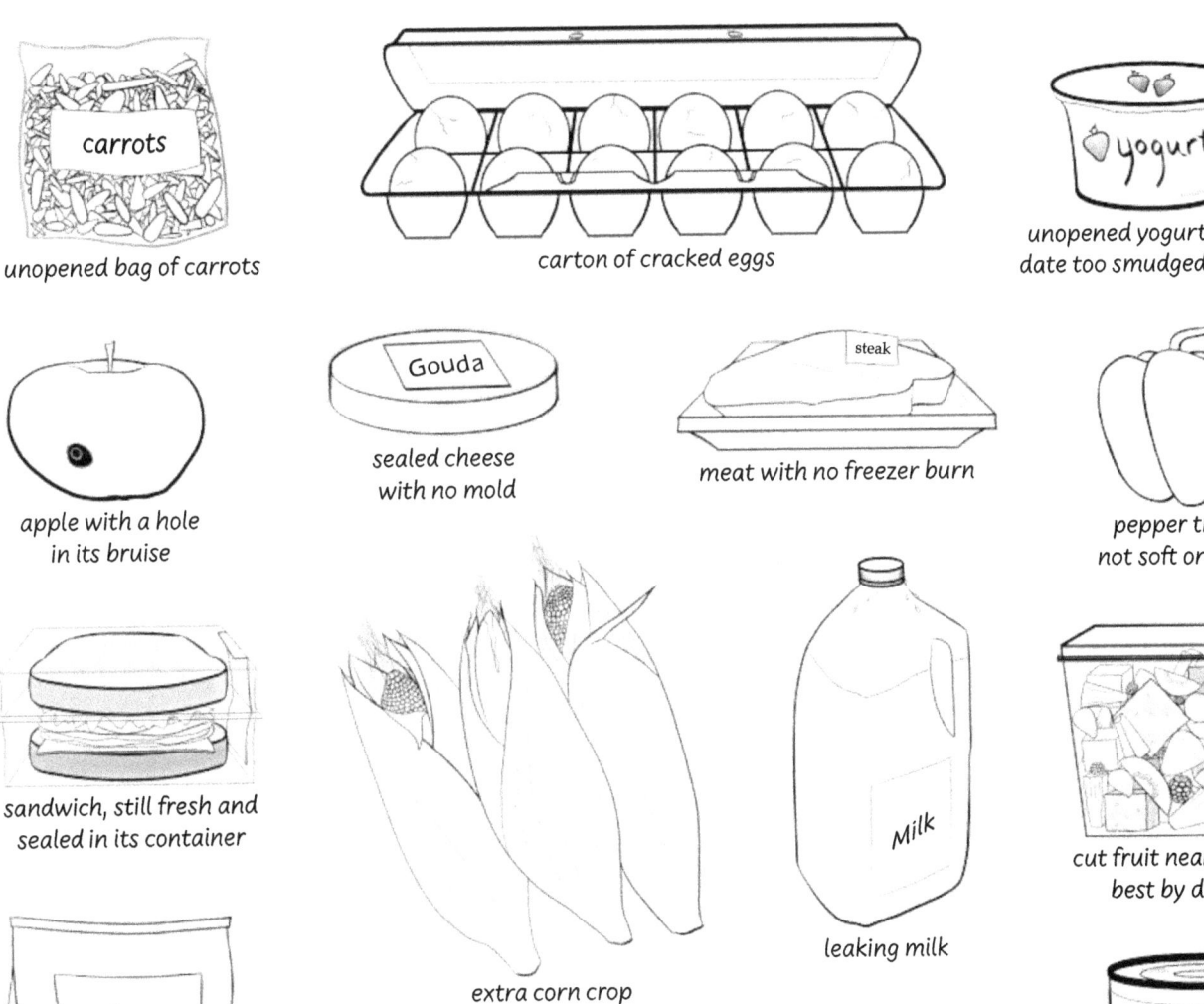

unopened bag of carrots

carton of cracked eggs

unopened yogurt with a date too smudged to read

apple with a hole in its bruise

sealed cheese with no mold

meat with no freezer burn

pepper that is not soft or moldy

sandwich, still fresh and sealed in its container

extra corn crop

leaking milk

cut fruit nearing its best by date

unopened bulk flour

bread that has started to mold

can with its label torn off

black bean can with a small dent

You took on the role of a food bank volunteer in that activity, giving your time to do service of that kind. As you were looking at the imaginary food bank's new supply of food, you only had a little information and your thoughts to guide you. It probably wasn't too hard, but volunteers have a lot of help to be sure.

For example, food bank workers train and help volunteers by:

⟶ saying what needs to be on food labels (and still be readable, too).

⟶ setting what dates (sell by, use by, best by...) are accepted each day.

⟶ showing how to know what has spoiled and/or become unsafe.

⟶ giving a list of items that cannot be accepted even if they are good.

⟶ directing how to box the food for the next stage.

⟶ being there to answer any questions.

Food banks need the help of volunteers to be able to sort more food and have less spoil in the process. Sound like a lot of work? I've not even shared everything employees do to keep food banks running well!

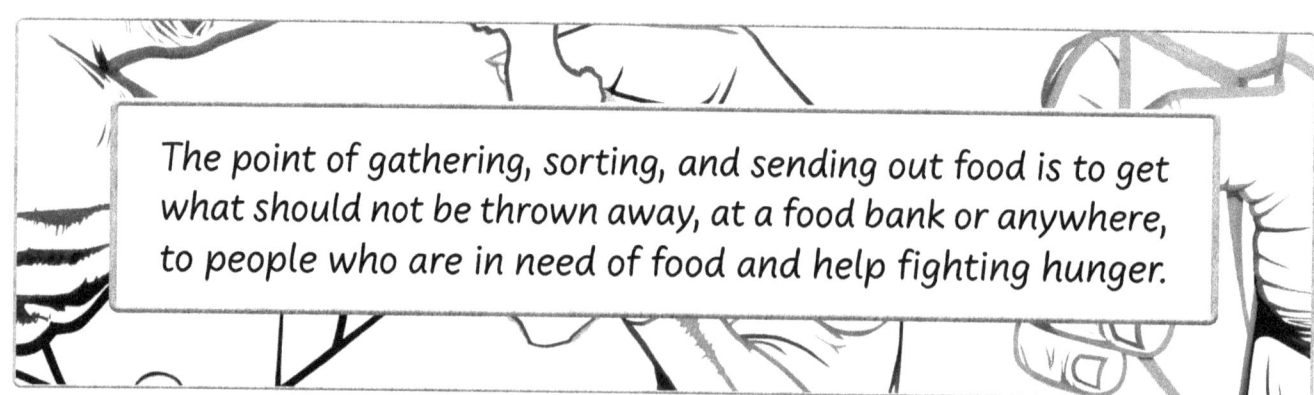

The point of gathering, sorting, and sending out food is to get what should not be thrown away, at a food bank or anywhere, to people who are in need of food and help fighting hunger.

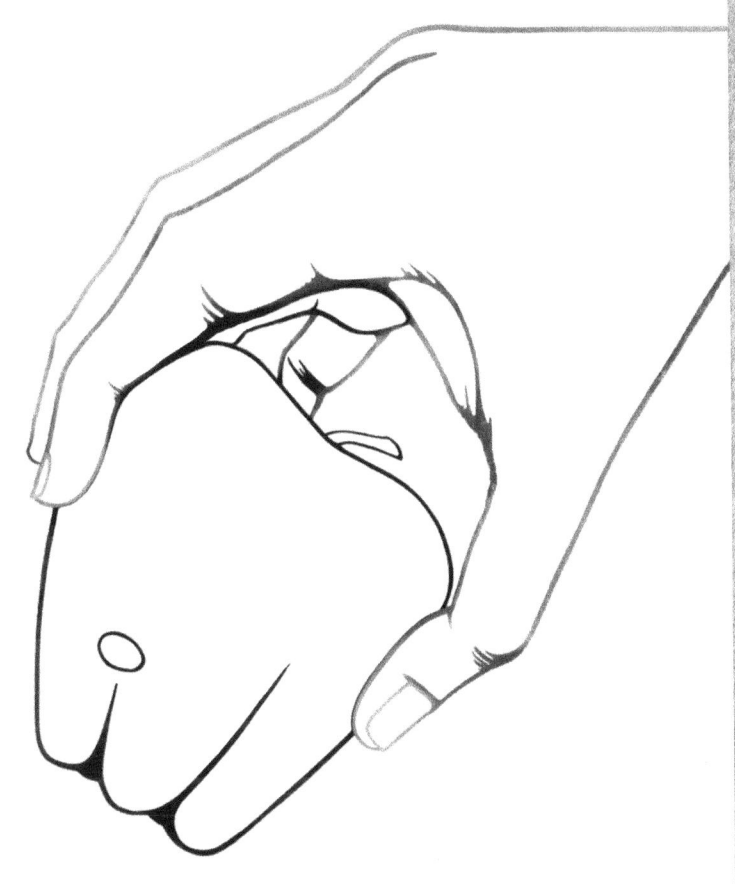

For each person's health,

whole grains, proteins, and produce

are the most needed fare,

which needn't be perfect, but good and safe,

for all to eat with food to spare.

Good food, then, gets sent out to more sites

—churches, food pantries and soup kitchens, among other places—

where serving people is one of their chief missions.

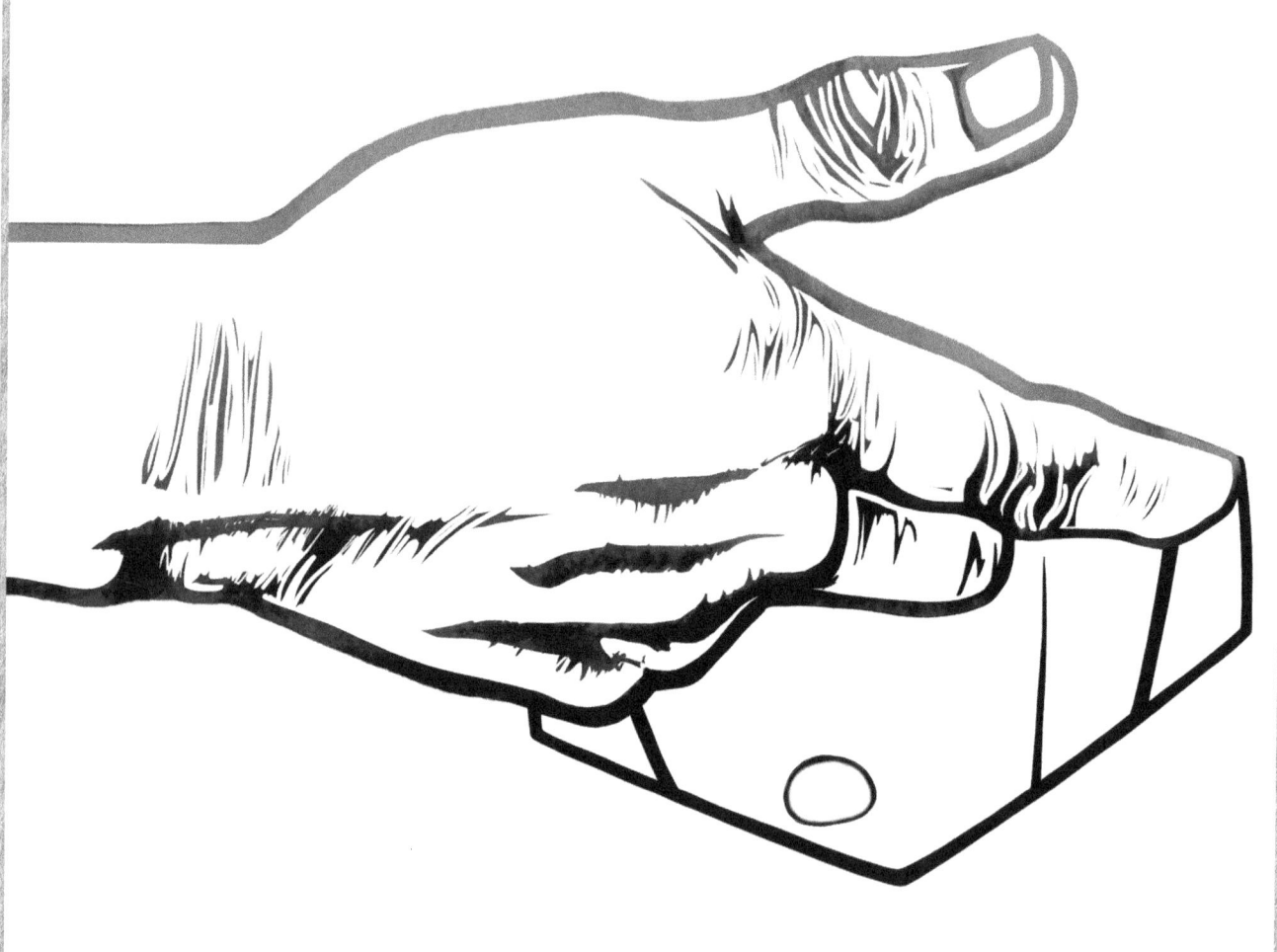

Find all the food and drink names you can! There are 50.
(See page 14 if you want to know what words to look for.)

S	J	K	S	P	I	N	A	C	H	H	U	J	C	O
A	A	A	T	J	A	M	P	T	P	A	P	A	Y	A
L	P	L	R	E	W	A	T	E	R	M	E	L	O	N
S	P	E	A	C	H	V	B	E	A	N	S	A	G	P
A	L	P	W	D	T	O	F	U	L	S	T	P	U	A
P	E	I	B	R	O	C	C	O	L	I	O	E	R	S
O	S	T	E	A	K	A	H	Y	A	M	M	N	T	T
T	E	A	R	D	T	D	K	I	W	I	A	O	O	A
A	M	O	R	I	C	O	R	N	C	L	T	Y	R	M
T	A	F	I	S	H	B	B	G	E	K	O	T	T	I
O	N	I	E	H	U	Y	R	E	R	Z	E	U	I	S
E	G	G	S	E	M	R	D	E	E	A	S	N	L	O
S	O	A	T	S	M	I	V	P	A	F	P	A	L	K
K	L	E	T	T	U	C	E	G	L	D	P	E	A	R
P	C	H	E	E	S	E	B	A	N	A	N	A	S	A

Food and Drink List:

1. apples	7. broccoli	13. fig	19. jam	25. miso	31. pear	37. rice	44. tofu
2. avocado	8. cereal	14. fish	20. kale	26. oats	32. peas	38. salad	45. tomatoes
3. bananas	9. cheese	15. grapes	21. kiwi	27. okra	33. pesto	39. salsa	46. tortillas
4. beans	10. chicken	16. ham	22. lettuce	28. papaya	34. pita	40. spinach	47. tuna
5. beef	11. corn	17. hummus	23. mango	29. pasta	35. potatoes	41. steak	48. watermelon
6. bread	12. eggs	18. jalapeño	24. milk	30. peach	36. radishes	42. strawberries	49. yam
						43. tea	50. yogurt

Gather the numbers on the path that makes it all the way through.

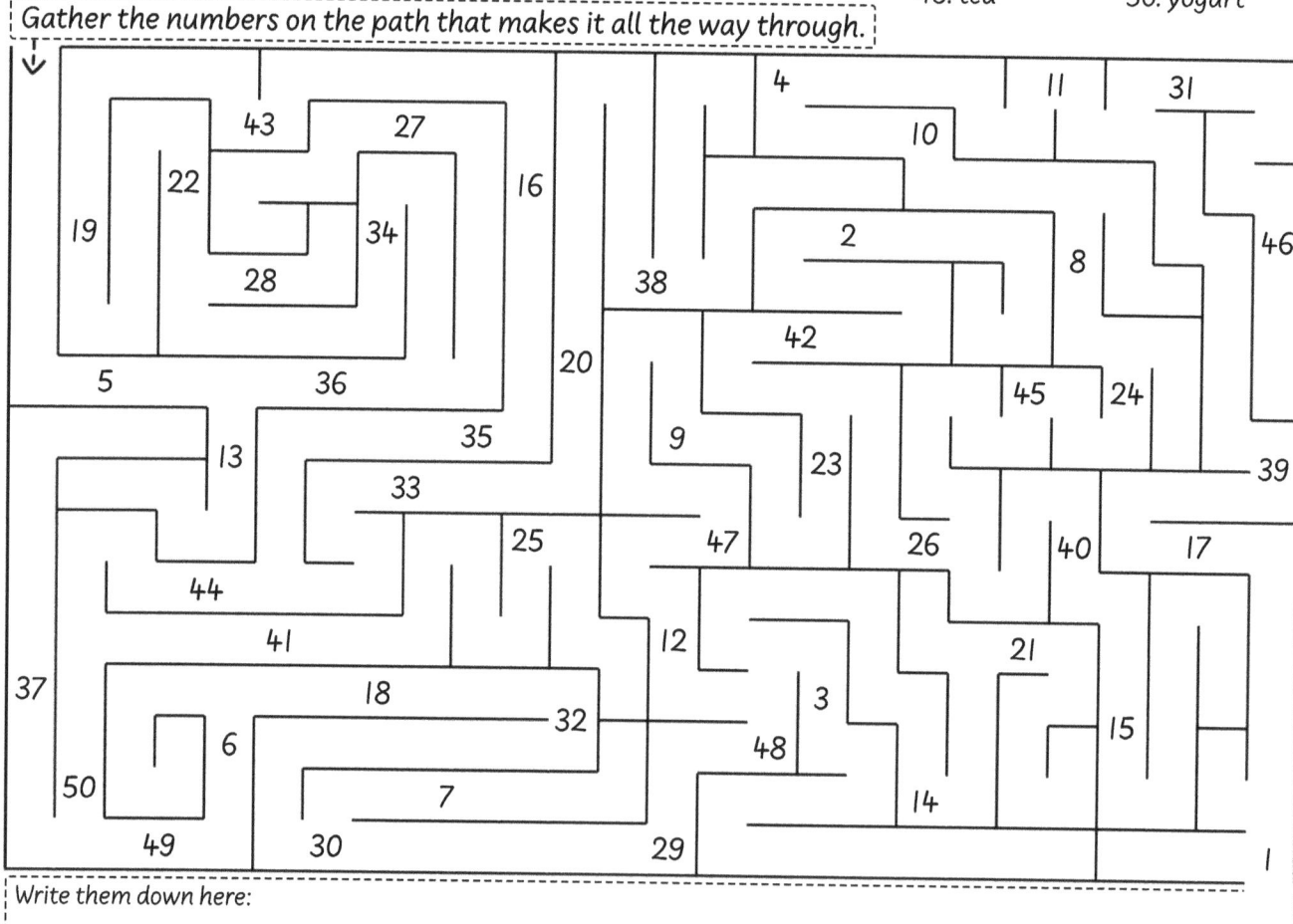

Write them down here:

Using the numbers you just gathered and the list of food, plan a meal or a whole day's meals.

Those activities' items are just examples of what could be at food pantries. Real food help places differ from this and from one another in the types of things and amounts available due to the size of their space, their sources of support, and other factors. More ways they might differ include:

- whether or not refrigerated or frozen items can be offered.
- whether their stock has set items or options that could change from time to time.
- how people get the food, from box deliveries or pick-ups to going and choosing.
- what, if any, terms or conditions they have for people to share in what's offered.
- open hours and how often one can get more food supplies.

Disaster, bad crops, high food prices,
low income, job loss, unemployment:
near despair, with no money to spare,
some make choices like eat or pay rent.

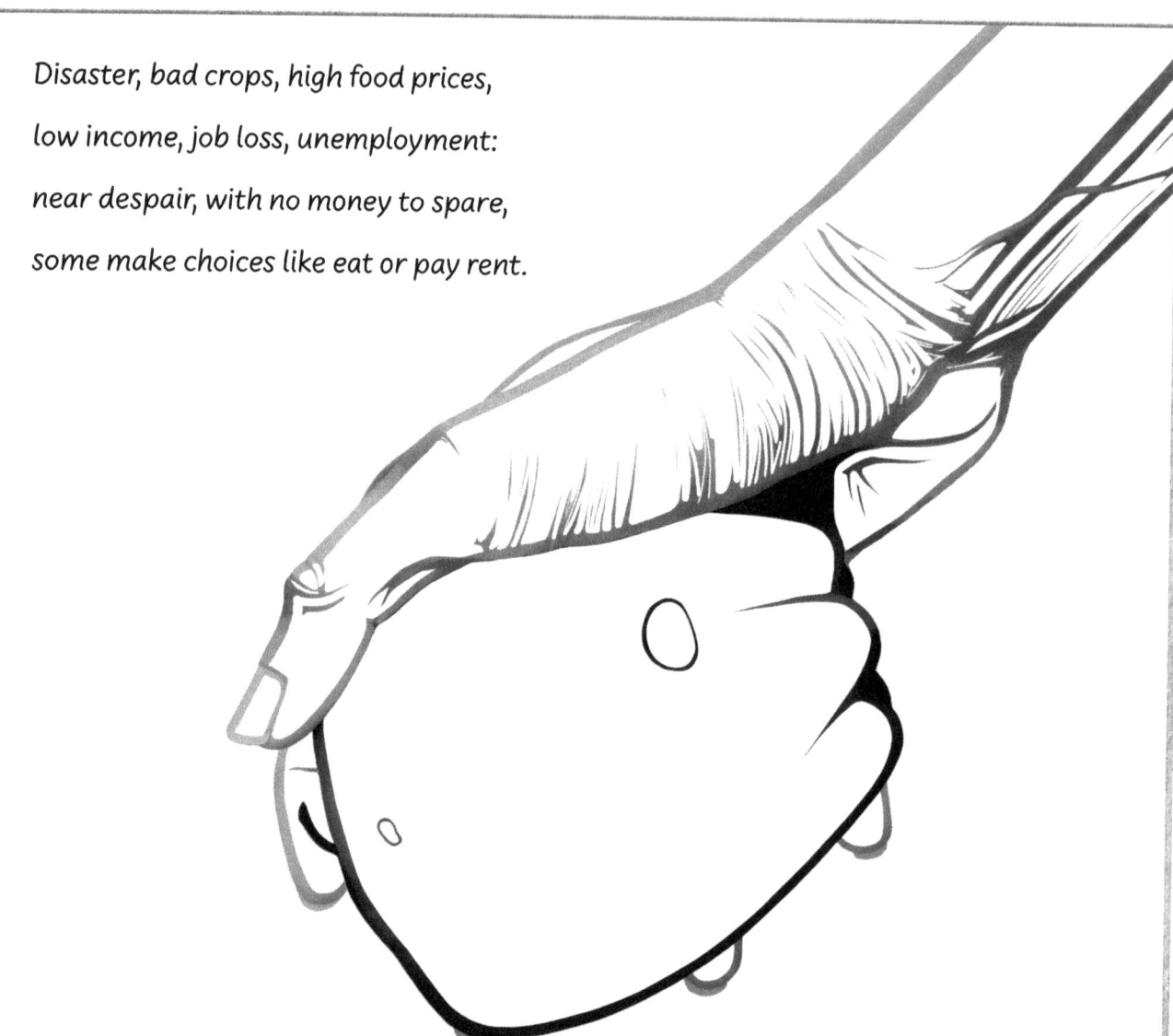

We've all felt the slight pangs of hunger that come before many of our meals,
but hunger takes over when it stays—moods, focus, health and futures, it steals.

Food needs are terribly relentless. How long would your planned meal keep you full?

Draw someone you would not want to be going without enough daily food.

You may have drawn a type of person, like a kid, but many of you have likely drawn someone you know, like a family member or a friend, your teacher or a classmate. That makes total sense...you know and care about them! As for anyone who's a stranger to you, they may be the person someone else drew or would draw if asked to do this sketch too. In truth, I know one who would draw you, and me, and every person.

Everyone matters, yet, all over the world, countless go hungry or go through a daily struggle of not knowing whether they will have anything to eat for their next meal. Thinking about these things can bring up a lot of hard questions, like the following ones. These are shared just to stress how complex hunger is and to show you that you're not alone in wrestling with it. You do not have to answer them.

Why is there so much hunger in the world? Why does even one person go hungry?

Why are they hungry/why am I hungry while we/others have plenty of food each day?

Should I get help? Can I handle this?

Is there anyone they/we/I can trust?

Will people look down on me for getting help?

Does anyone understand?

Why do some have contempt for people in need? Do I?

Should help only be for those who don't deserve what they're going through?
Is that how the world works? Is that how we want it to work? Should it work that way?

Does this or that way of help make a difference? Or does it keep them/us/me stuck?

What help gets down to the roots?

What's the right thing to do?

Why won't [whoever] do anything?

Is part of the problem that people just don't care enough? Or, that not enough people care?

Is there a way to bring about good
without forcing people?

Is it even possible to rid the world of hunger?

For stopping life-consuming hunger, one must face down every root problem,

or, while we help meet urgent needs, it will persist through what's at its bottom.

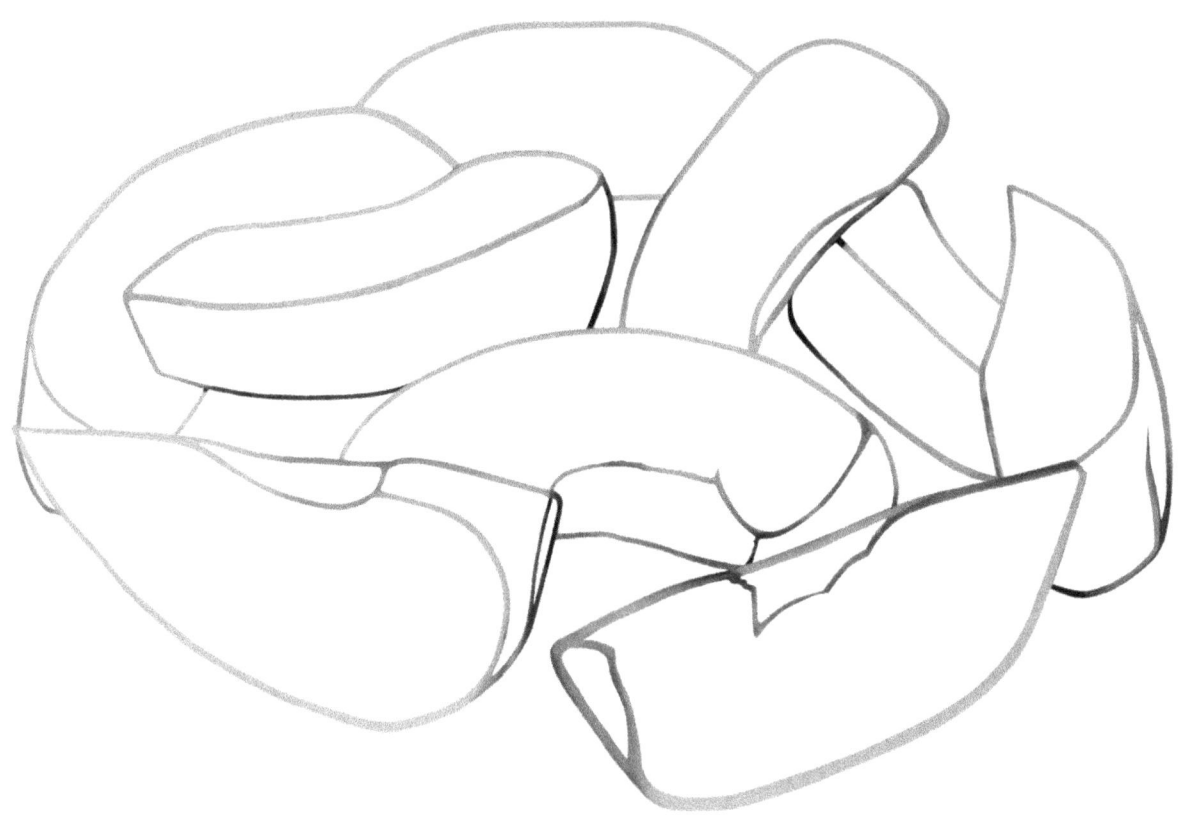

But food banks do help lighten the hold hunger has, making things more stable

until the gap is gone between what people have and need on their table.

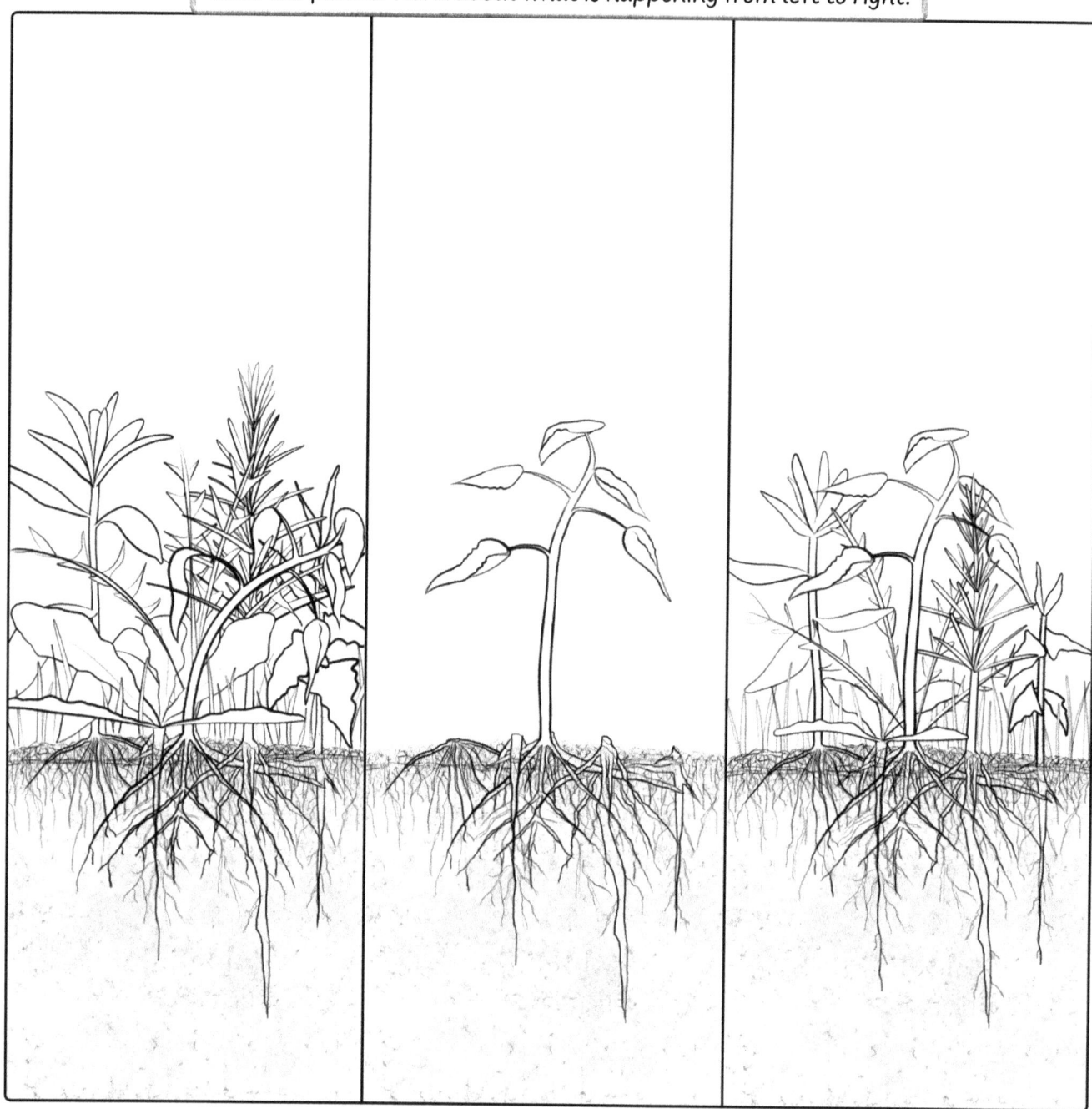

20

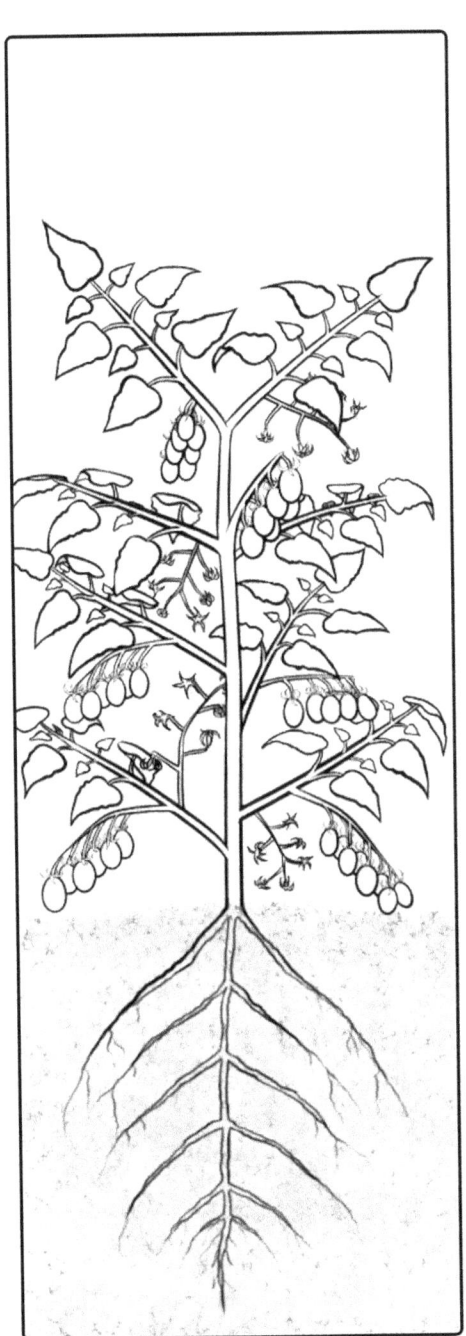

Unmet food needs cause increasing harm, much like weeds do, so the help provided by food assistance places and programs is vital, yet this help, by itself, is like removing weeds solely above the soil surface. This gives real relief, but it's always short-term. Why? The remaining roots keep growing more weeds. Similarly, every cause of hunger must be dealt with to end it completely.

But, unlike how we can usually dig up weed roots with relative simplicity, needing only a tool, some strength, and a bit of time, truly ending every cause of hunger is not that straightforward. And if there is even just one root cause left remaining, one issue in the plan or operation of any of the solutions, one new cause of hunger that existing solutions cannot prevent or address, then hunger cannot be ended for all and especially not forevermore.

There are many things we might hope in to end hunger...upright leaders, laws, policies, and practices; well-managed resources; learning and work opportunities for all; fair wages; agricultural advancements; conflict resolution; affordable basic necessities; unity and more. These all have the potential for positive impacts and should be pursued in good and wise ways, but can they be our hope for a complete global and permanent end of hunger?

Which of those, alone or even all together, can be achieved and impact the entire world at once? Which of those is guaranteed to last? What can end evil? What can bring about true peace and justice, with mercy for anyone who seeks it? And what about the things our food supply is vulnerable to, like the weather, that we ultimately cannot control? Moreover, what can do anything real and lasting within our hearts, concerning our hardness and the weeds of wrongness (laziness, greed, self-centeredness, and so on)? And what can stop the devastation of diseases and death?

Are we hopeless? Looking at these, yes. But there is good news.

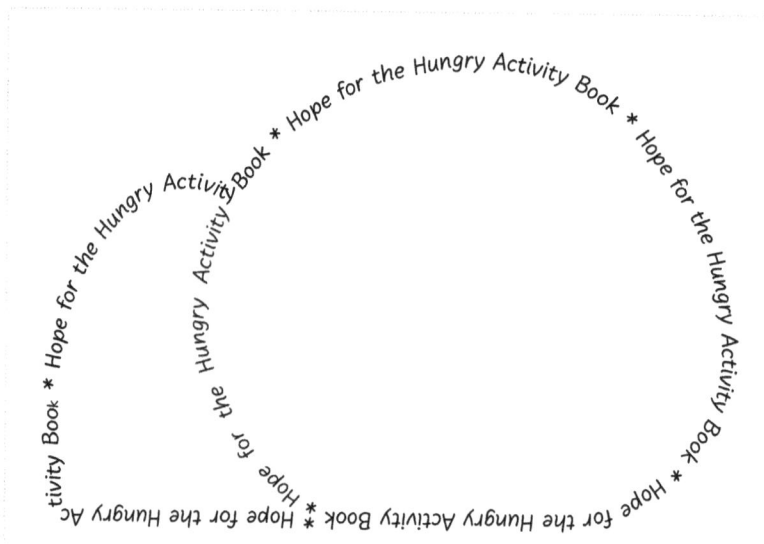

Hope for the Hungry Activity Book * Hope for the Hungry Activity Book * Hope for the Hungry Activity Book * Hope for the Hungry Activity Book * Hope for the Hungry Activity Book

Looking to the Word of God

We may think that the reality of hunger means that God is not real, or maybe that He doesn't care or that He's not able to handle it. In view of or experiencing actual suffering, that is easy to believe. At one time, I did. But, let me now share the good news with you! Here is the truth—the truth that stands up to all of the hunger, suffering and evil in the world, the truth that will wipe them out completely and permanently.

HERE IS HOPE

There is one who has and will come in power whose glorious reign will never end. And this one I speak of is truly good and kind and just. He redeems and saves, provides for, protects, guides and walks closely with all of His people. He is attentive and compassionate, holy and patient and wise; loving and loved by all of His people. Who is this? Our Creator; God; the Messiah. The one who has given us our very lives gave His own to guarantee new life in this Kingdom for anyone who comes to belong to Him by His grace. When God brings this Kingdom to fulfillment, there will be no more suffering, crying, pain, or death. That is unimaginably good! But how can that truly be? By God keeping all of His Holy Spirit-given promises through His Son, the Lord Jesus Christ. How can we be sure He will? Because Jesus did die for all of us, and yet He does not simply live on in memory; Jesus rose from the dead on the third day, as He said He would, and is seated by God the Father. One day, all will know He is Lord. Until then, the eternal, unchanging God makes Himself known to us by His Word and Spirit so that we may believe and enter His Kingdom by the salvation He gives.

Don't just take my word for it. Come, see and hear for yourself!

From here on, I'll be sharing verses from the Bible, the Word of God. I hope you find and read them. They're on the internet, on apps, and in print. Take your time reading! It's a lot, but always worth it. Use whatever translation you have access to. For some activities, you may have to look up another.

Let's learn how to find verses in a printed Bible and practice with Revelation 21: 3 - 7.

(Title) Use the table of contents to turn to the page number for the indicated book. Find Revelation. (#:) The bold, bigger numbers that mark various sections are the chapter numbers. Find that 21. (:#s) The smaller numbers within the writing are the verse numbers. Read verses 3, 4, 5, 6, and 7!

(longest one) Genesis 1~3 — Hunger is one result of the _____ people from _____ with God. Sin entices and ensnares us to be without care for what _____.

Jeremiah 2:17 and 4:18 — God wants us to follow Him because He is good and sin _____. Still, we often reject God's way _____ and _____.

Ephesians 2:1~13 — While we are still sinners who do not belong to God by faith in Jesus Christ, we are _____ and, being _____, we are _____.

Proverbs 19:15 — Not all who _____ are idle, but those who _____ will hunger. God has warned us that a _____ is suffering hunger.

2 Thessalonians 3:6~13 — Sometimes _____ Christ-believers too. Being _____ work is wrong. God commands us all to be _____ with our lives.

Isaiah 10:1~2 — Much suffering comes from the _____ that disregard God's will, keeping poor people _____, and robbed _____.

1 Peter 5:8 — The devil, who got Eve and Adam to _____ God, is still on the _____ to _____—especially believers' (as much as he can).

Job 1:6~22 — Suffering is not always a result of the _____. It can be from _____ uses loss, suffering, and death _____ make us hate God.

Ephesians 6:10~12 — A force of _____ carries out dark plans. Our _____ them. In Christ, we may stand in the _____ God.

Lamentations 3:19~33 — God may_____ suffering because our greatest need is to turn to God, to have real faith and _____ Him and wait for His _____.

Philippians 4:10~13 — Whatever we go through, God gives His people _____ and helps us learn _____ as He proves He is faithful and trustworthy in _____.

Hebrews 12:3~11 — Hardships may be _____ God, who _____ things to bring about _____ in and for His children.

1 Peter 1:1~9 — Trials _____ is truly real. And, by God's power and grace, our _____ in _____ as Christ is revealed. Praise God!

Romans 8:31~39 — Since we _____ by Christ's _____, believers suffer for the _____, that all people might know Christ Jesus.

Can anyone but God forgive and end sin, give new life, destroy evil, and work everything in this life for our eternal good?

all that we face

of their rights

bring about or allow

prowl looking

separated from God

saving grace

are hungry

glory and honor

loving discipline from

are idle

His strength

endure and overcome

without hope

poor, struggling

is destructive

prove one's faith

power and protection of

productive and helpful

to try to

glory of God

unwilling to

suffer the consequences

actions of leadership

fellowship and life

trials may result

destructive result of idleness

for our way

good transformations

spiritual evil

sufferer having sinned

works in all

idleness ensnares

destroy lives

without God

the devil, who

fall of

turn their backs on

struggle is against

will result of it

presence, power, and love

to be content

hope in

Not having much or any suffering in one's life is not proof of being in right standing with God.
see Psalm 73

God's command that the poor be cared for does not give anyone a right to idly rely on this care. While some do that, be mindful that many who want to work have trials getting or keeping a job and many work for merely enough or for less than they need. Willingness is not known by money.
see 2 Thessalonians 3:6~10 *and* James 5:1~6

Whoever truly believes in Christ Jesus will never be forsaken [left alone and helpless] by God, thus a believer's suffering never means God has taken away His love and power. God is faithful.
see Hebrews 13:5~6

God Himself creates some of the world's suffering, but it always advances His plan of salvation and never goes against His Word or honor. It is vital that our understanding of God is from the truth of who He is, as revealed by His Spirit in His Word. Otherwise, we make up who we think He is and what He's like based on our lives and feelings. Such thoughts fall terribly short of the truth.
see Isaiah 45

The existence of suffering does not mean God is not able to deal with and end it. Keep reading!
see Luke 1

That the world has suffering does not mean God's enemies are beating Him or His good plans.
see Luke 18:31~43

Allowing people to sin and His enemies to carry on with evil does not make any of it God's fault. Yes, God is the Most High. But God will never force anyone to trust, love, and follow Jesus Christ.
see James 1:12~15

God will end suffering, but it is also for our good that God waits. We will look at this again later.
see 2 Peter 3:8~10

Now let's go back to the weeds in us. What do you take in daily to feed your mind, heart, and soul? The things of school or work, entertainment, and social media? We have been given much to learn, do, and enjoy, but we must be careful what we let shape us and grow in us. What happens to us when those things that fill and lead our lives have no real care for God or even clearly hate Him? Among other things, we starve spiritually. Read Matthew 4:1-11, with special focus on verse four. May God expose and uproot everything harmful and feed you life-giving truth. Read Psalm 34:8!

True or False:

Make your best guesses before turning the page!

_____ The Bible was written under the complete authority of God, that people might believe and live by faith.

Through the Holy Bible:

_____ We may come to know God.

_____ We hear of what God has done in the past and will do in the future.

_____ We learn that God has set a final day for judgment.

_____ We are convicted—we find out we are guilty of sinning against [defying/doing wrong to] God.

_____ We find out that we will be alright if we just try our best to be good and keep God's law.

_____ We learn that if we go to church we will be saved.

_____ We hear that God loves us and sent Jesus Christ—the only one who can make us right with God.

_____ We find out that Jesus died in our place and that He is alive and on the throne in heaven.

_____ We hear that God gives salvation through Jesus Christ to whoever believes in Him [the Son of God].

_____ We know that since God gives us full forgiveness through Christ, we can do whatever we want.

_____ We are assured that life will be easy for us once we believe and become God's children.

_____ God gives His people comfort, guidance, strength, hope and so much more.

The Bible was written under the complete authority of God, that people might believe and live by faith.
True. See John 20:30~31, 2 Timothy 3:14~17, and 2 Peter 1:16~21.

1. We may come to know God.

    True. See Hebrews 1:1~3, Hebrews 13:8, and John 14:6~7.

2. We hear of what God has done in the past and will do in the future.

    True. See Exodus 14:1~18, Isaiah 48:3~5, Hebrews 6:13~20, and 2 Peter 3:1~7.

3. We learn that God has set a final day for judgment.

    True. See Isaiah 66:14~16, Acts 17:30~31, and Hebrews 4:13.

4. We are convicted—we find out we are guilty of sinning against [defying/doing wrong to] God.

    True. See Isaiah 53:6, Romans 1:16~23, and Romans 3:9~23.

5. We find out that we will be alright if we just try our best to be good and keep God's law.

    False. See Luke 18:9~14, Galatians 3:10~12, Romans 7:7~24, and Titus 3:3~8. Desiring to obey God and doing good by faith in Christ is different than trusting in ourselves for being found righteous in God's judgment.

6. We learn that if we go to church we will be saved.

    False. All believers belong in the Church, but people can be with the Church regularly and yet never have faith in Jesus Christ. See Matthew 7:21~23, Hebrews 4:1~2, Jude 1:3~4, Colossians 2:18~23, and John 3:3.

7. We hear that God loves us and sent Jesus Christ—the only one who can make us right with God.

    True. See John 1:29, 3:36 & 14:6; Acts 4:11~12; Ephesians 2:1~13; Colossians 2:8~15; & 1 Timothy 2:1~6.

8. We find out that Jesus died in our place and that He is alive and on the throne in heaven.

    True! See Isaiah 53, Matthew 26~28:10, 1 Corinthians 15:3~7, Hebrews 1:1~3 and 9:23~28.

9. We hear that God gives salvation through Jesus Christ to whoever believes in Him [the Son of God].

    True! See John 1:9~14, 3:16 & 5:24; Acts 10:43; Romans 3:21~26 & 6:23; and Hebrews 7:18~25.

10. We know that since God gives us full forgiveness through Christ, we can do whatever we want.

    False. God does fully forgive His people, but, by faith, Christ Jesus is also our Lord whom we now love and thus begin to obey out of love. See Romans 8:1~14, Galatians 5:13~26, 1 Peter 1:13~25, and 1 John 1:5~2:6.

11. We are assured that life will be easy for us once we believe and become God's children.

    False. See John 16:33, Romans 5:1~5, Romans 8:14~39, 1 Peter 4:12~19, and 1 John 5:4~5.

12. God gives His people comfort, guidance, strength, hope and so much more.

    True! See 2 Corinthians 1:3~5, John 10:14~16, Psalm 23, John 14:15~31, and Ephesians 1:2~14.

I encourage you to read each of those verses and passages, even when you got the answer right!
Notes and reflections:

Why read? God says faith comes from hearing the Word of God, the message of Jesus Christ (see Romans 10:17). That's so good and simple! As you read, though, keep in mind that we can read without paying attention, we can listen for what we want to hear, we can carry on as if the message doesn't really matter...we can, but these are warning signs of not believing. In truth, without God calling us to Jesus and giving us genuine faith in Him, none of us would believe (see John 5:39 - 40). Spiritual evil blinds us, sin hardens our hearts, and Jesus' cross even confronts our belief that we're good enough. How good that God desires our salvation! God opens our ears to truly hear, our minds to see Jesus' glory, and our hearts to receive Him (see 2 Corinthians 4:6), so that, by God's grace, we who've lived as intentional or unknowing enemies of God are brought to peace with God and new life in Christ (see Romans 5:1 - 11 and 1 Peter 1:3 - 5). Jesus will never cast out anyone who comes to Him in faith (see John 6:37).

In John 8:58, Jesus made a momentous statement about Himself, restating a revelation in Exodus 3. Let's hear seven more "I am" statements Jesus made about core truths He wants us to know of Him. The spiral below has the first letter of each word. Read everything that Jesus said and fill in the rest!

John 6:35, 48; John 8:12; John 10:7, 9; John 10:11-18; John 11:25; John 14:6; John 15:1, 5
(Look up the English Standard Version, the American Standard Version, or the New King James Version for John 10:7, 9.)

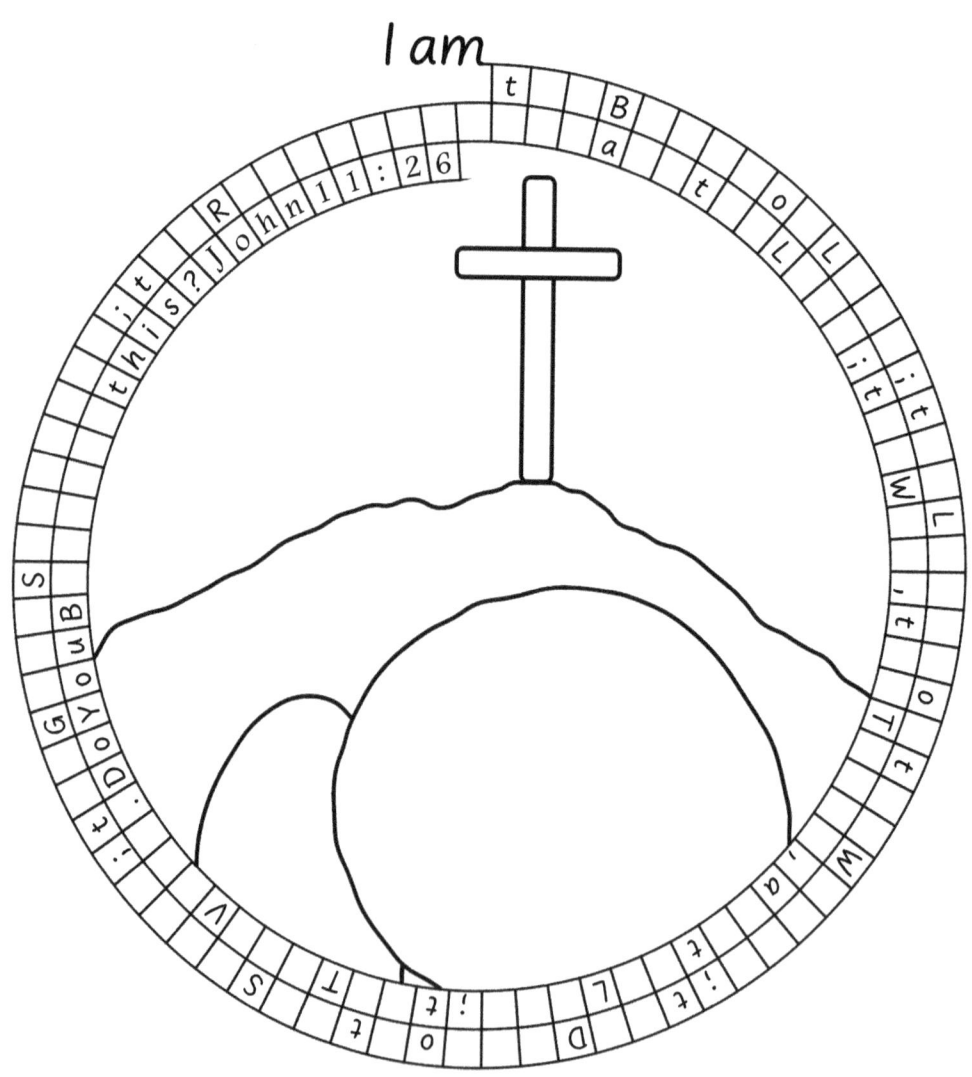

I am

God's Plan of Love

Hands are a visual theme of these books, but the ones that I hope you take to heart are the hands that are not drawn here. These are, markedly, God's hands.

Read Isaiah 49:16.

This is one of the times that God told us, hundreds of years ahead of time, what Jesus would do for us. And not just that, God is saying it means we can trust Him that He will never forget or forsake His people. How can we know that so confidently? Because the eternal Son of God was sent and willingly came to be born fully human, yet fully God: God in flesh; God With Us...tempted and tried, yet absolutely triumphant (see Hebrews 4:15 & John 8:28-29!)...and, as planned, He went to the cross for us (see 1 Peter 2:22-25). When Jesus Christ was nailed through his hands to save us, He engraved us on the palms of His hands. He said He would and He did. God is truly faithful; He always keeps His Word, even hundreds of years later, even when doing so meant He would suffer and die.

Read Romans 5:8 again.

Why is it vital that Jesus gave Himself up for us? Read Romans 6:23 again.

Before creating people, God made death to be the price for sin. What's more, prior to physical death, we're already spiritually dead in our sins and are unable to raise ourselves to life. We each deserve the wrath that God has in store for all unrighteousness. But God, because of His great love for us, provided a way for justice to be upheld and mercy given. The Son of God laid His life down by taking on our flesh to reign over it with perfect love for the Father and a sinless life and, then, by taking our sin in His body to the cross, where He nailed it and paid our price by His own blood and death. Jesus was truly sinless; He did not have to die. He would not have died ever. And, being God, having all authority, no one could take His life from Him. Jesus was killed only as He gave Himself up to fulfill the plan made by God the Father, Son, and Spirit before our creation—before we even needed salvation. This is the sacrifice that God planned, promised and pointed to: the lifeblood of God for our forgiveness and eternal life. Our hope of salvation rests in the glorious truth that God raised Jesus from the grave to heaven's throne. Jesus' sacrifice was proven accepted! Thus, with life, God gives righteousness to whoever receives the Lord Jesus Christ: any before Him who lived by faith in God and His promise to send a Messiah for our salvation and any after His coming who believes that Jesus is the promised Messiah and Risen Lord. Jesus engraved us on the palms of His hands to give His life for us and to us; He will never forsake us. For all who repent and believe the good news of Christ, God's life is the gift and guarantee of salvation.

What word is meant by each cryptic message?

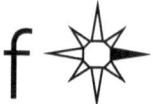   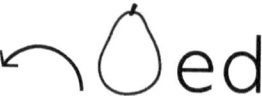   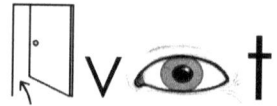

_____   _____   _____

Thankfully, God's plans and His expressed desire for us to be in them are much more clear in His Word!

Let's take a look at one related to hunger and its promised end.

WHAT? From Isaiah 25:6 - 9 and Revelation 21:1 - 8, describe the celebration and life God has promised.

These verses give a general picture of what's promised, of the glory to come, but we truly can't imagine all the good that God has planned for those who will inherit His Kingdom through and with Jesus Christ.

WHEN? Well, we don't quite know when...but other promises of God help us wait in patient hope for this. Here's one we have already looked at in part: read John 14:1 - 7. What did Jesus say, particularly in 1 - 3?

Also, read 1 Corinthians 15. What does it have to do with the great banquet God promised in Isaiah 25?

WHO? Who is invited? And who will be there? The most simple answer is in John 3:16. What is written?

GOD
ISAIAH 55:11
THE THRONE OF GRACE, HEAVEN

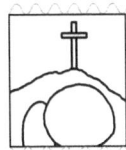

God does not mail invitations from heaven, but He definitely gives them to us!
Read Isaiah 55 and 2 Corinthians 5:11-21.

Whether sent directly or through a messenger, invitations come from the host. Invitations are personal, showing that we are wanted, and they are a vital link between the plan and our presence when it's time, giving us the opening and responsibility to decide. Getting invited somewhere may move us to go, or not. Have you ever been invited to something, yet not go? I hope none of us put off or reject God's invitation. One day, the wait will be over. For now, God is giving us time to respond to Him. Remember 2 Peter 3:9? As Jesus says in Matthew 22:1-14, many will refuse. But what does that hard part about clothes mean?

The wedding clothes are symbolic of salvation through Jesus Christ.
See Isaiah 61, Luke 4:14-21, Isaiah 1:18, John 1:29, Romans 3:21-26, Revelation 7:13-17 and 20:11-21:8.

God invites us to come through His Son Jesus, the Door of the Sheep; open to all, but the only way. Why? Not entering through Christ (so not being clothed in the garments of salvation) is going in our sinfulness instead of in His righteousness. Sin destroys life but God has promised peace; thus, anyone who wants to remain a sinner, who rejects Jesus Christ as their Savior and/or refuses His Lordship, will not be welcome. How does Jesus invite us to God's Kingdom in Mark 1:15? (Also, see Luke 24:44-47 and Acts 2:36-39.)

What does that word mean?...To see sin as it truly is and be turned away from it, to want forgiven of it and saved from it, and to not make a practice of it anymore all by turning to Jesus Christ through faith in Him. Repentance itself does not save us, God does, but it is an essential part of believing what we have heard and it is a result of God's grace in our lives. See Acts 11:11-18. What is your response to God's invitation?

Describe what our Creator wants life to be like for us and for all of His creation. Why isn't it that way?

Now, imagine if God treated sin as if it does not matter, as if everything is alright, as if we don't need to turn away from and be forgiven of anything just because He loves us. How could there be any hope of justice or even mercy; of true, lasting peace; of life without sorrow, pain and unending struggle?

Eternal life is not a mere carrying on of life as we know it—for God's people, it's joyful, abundant life with our loving and gracious God who will one day completely get rid of sin, suffering, evil, and death. But we are all sinners; we cannot live that life and we don't deserve it. In truth, because of our ways, living here and now in defiance of God and true good, we deserve the punishment of the eternal life God has warned us about—eternal separation from God, with no hope of redemption, goodness, help or relief. So eternal separation from God is not a carrying on of life as we know it either because, until it's the set time for judgment, God is gracious and patient with us, even when we are His enemies, and God is holding back, for now, the full horror and misery of being without Him and without hope. Dark though these days often still are, this time is for salvation. Because God loves us and is merciful and does not want us to die under our rightful condemnation, but, rather, wants us saved and with Him where He is forevermore, what has God promised? What has God done? Who and what is our hope?

Jesus does not save us once we have pleased God. He came, sent by God the Father, to seek and save sinners. And the sinners He saves, who receive the message and the Son of God Himself with belief, are redeemed and made a new, holy creation, forgiven and freed from darkness to live in God's light. Jesus will return as promised, yet His reign begins in our hearts the moment we repent and believe. Then, although salvation is not complete until He returns, we are in His Kingdom, safe in His hands. Hallelujah! See Romans 8:1, Ephesians 1:13~14, Philippians 1:6, Colossians 1:9~14, and Luke 12:32!

In Christ Crossword

Let's consider spiritual hunger again before we get back to physical hunger. Please read Matthew 5:6!

You can certainly fill in this crossword without every verse, but, as always, I recommend still reading all of them! That is so much better for you than just taking in the small taste of truth from my words. – May you be filled with hope!

1. God gives us right standing with Him when we've ___. See Romans 3:21~26.

2. Taken away. Our sins have been ___ by Jesus. See Psalm 103:11~12.

3. [↓] God makes ___ those seeking mercy, sorry for their sin. See Psalm 51.

3. [→] Jesus' righteousness put on us. We are ___. See Isaiah 61:10.

4. [↓] Receiving Christ, we're born again as God's ___. See John 1:9~13.

5. In Christ, we're rescued and have ___. See Colossians 1:9~14, 2:13~15.

6. [↓] God gives the Holy Spirit to dwell with us here: ___ us. See John 14:15~17.

7. God writes His law here for Jesus' people: on our ___. See Hebrews 8:10.

8. Children of God do not just have, but live by the ___. See Romans 8:1~17.

9. By Jesus' sacrifice once for all, His own are ___. See Hebrews 10:10~18.

10. By ___ we can have lives that are pleasing to God. See Hebrews 11:6~7.

11. After Christ saves us, He builds up godly lives by ___ us. See Titus 2:11~14.

12. [↓] We are free from sin's power, if under ___ in Christ. See Romans 6:1~14.

13. In thankfulness, from our hearts, we're willingly ___. See Romans 6:17.

14. Devoted to God and learning His Word, we are ___. See Romans 12:1~2.

15. The Spirit grows ___ in all who are Christ's. See Galatians 5:13~26.

16. God's discipline, in all who heed it, produces ___ too. See Hebrews 12:11.

17. God will ___ and purify all who confess their need for Christ. See 1 John 1:5~2:6.

18. [→] The righteous in Christ will live; the wicked will be ___ off. See Psalm 37.

19. By God's ___ we await the new creation of pure righteousness. See 2 Peter 3:13.

20. God will wipe away our ___ and put an end to suffering. See Revelation 21:1~8.

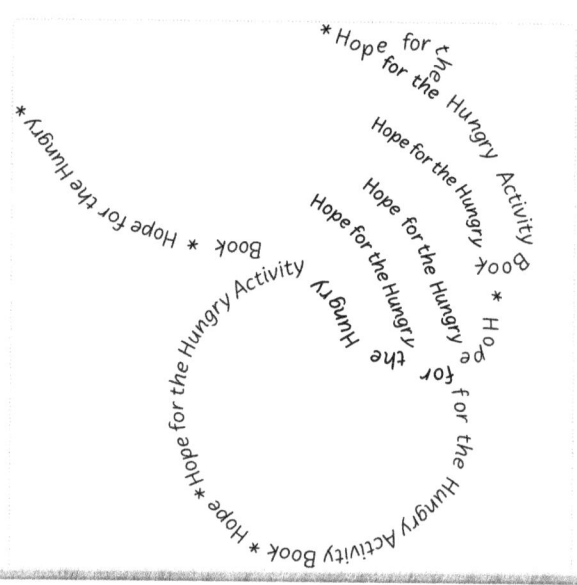

Our Faith Response

A hungerless world hasn't yet come—only Christ the Lord will achieve it—
but, while we wait, such good can be done
each time we give help or receive it.

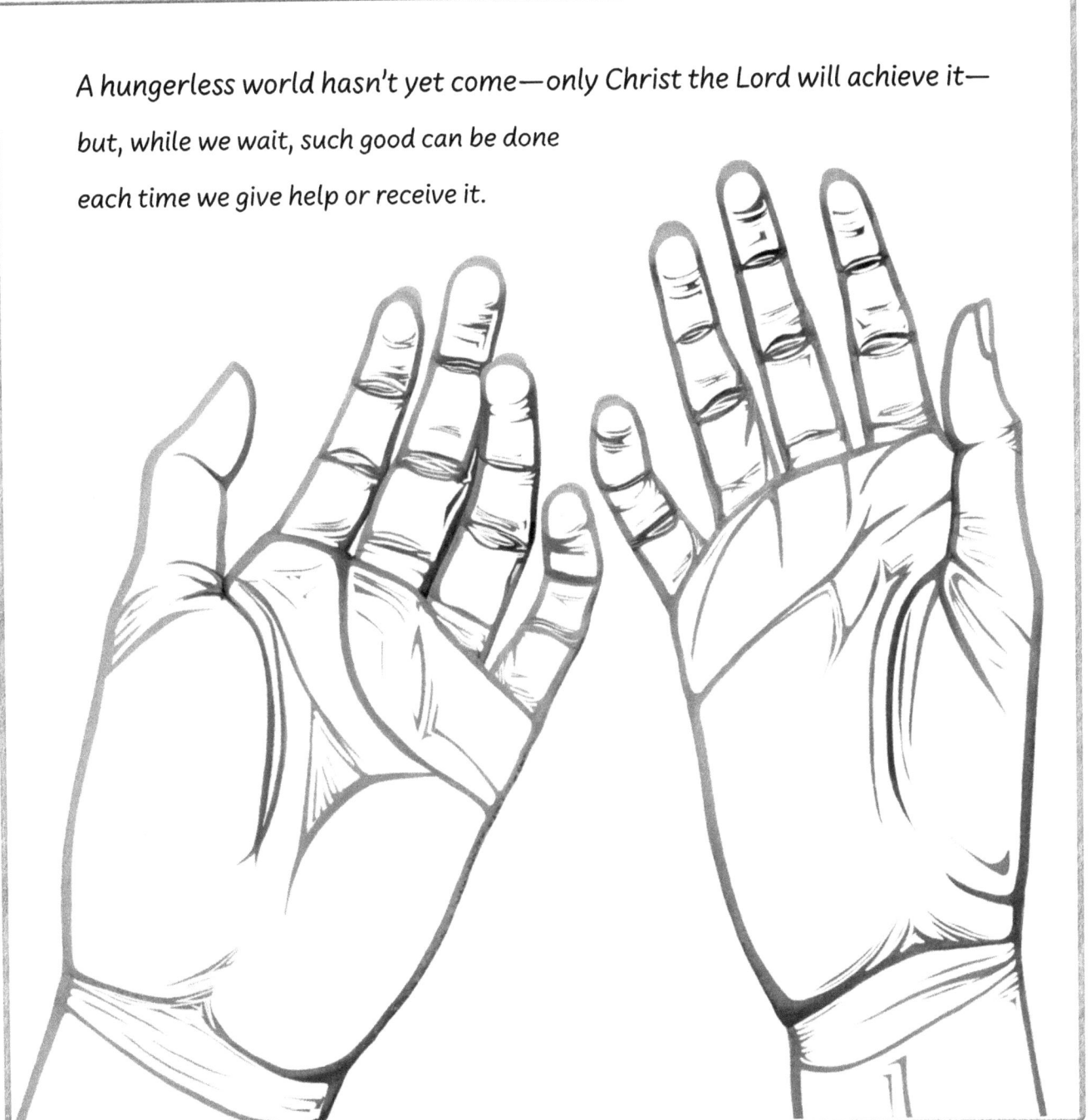

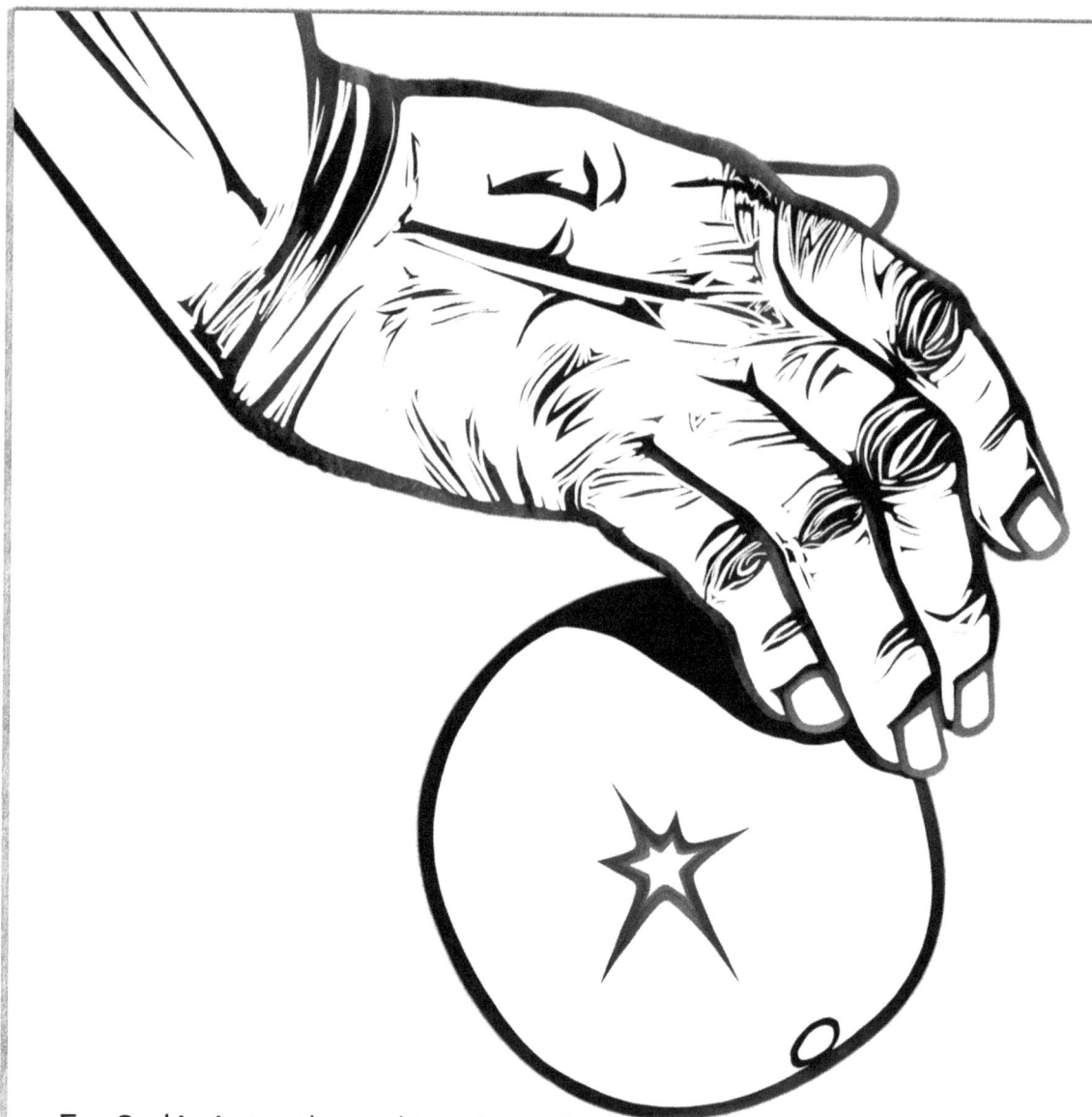

For God is, in truth, working through us with good works of His kindness and aid

to help His own and point to Jesus

until He meets each promise He made.

Draw lines to connect the right details in the following accounts.
Genesis 6:9~22; Genesis 37~50 (see 41:53~42:5); Exodus 16 & 17; Ruth (see chapters 1 & 2);
2 Samuel 9; 1 Kings 17:1~6; 1 Kings 17:7~24; 1 Kings 18:1~15; Daniel 1; and John 6:1~14.

God provided:	For:	Through:
bread and fish	the family and animals	Moses
vegetables and water	Elijah	David
bread and meat	Ruth and Naomi	Noah
grain from storehouses	the Widow at Zarephath and her son	a Guard
harvest gleanings, water, and bread	the Israelites	Ravens
food at the king's table, family land and its crops	Daniel, Hananiah, Mishael and Azariah	Joseph
manna, quail, and water	Prophets of the LORD	Elijah
continual flour and oil	the large crowd	Obadiah
every kind of food	Mephibosheth	Boaz
bread and water	Jacob's family	Jesus, a boy, and the disciples

That activity highlighted God's care and provision for people's physical needs. Sometimes God provided through acts of power and other times more simply through people's responses of active faith and care. But, no matter any differences in how the help was given, God always gave more than just food or water.

Connect the following blessings with the people from page 39 who also received them from God, then or later, through God's active provision for their physical needs. Use as many lines as you need here!

compassion [tender care in action]	Noah's family and the animals
kindness	Elijah
evidence of God's steadfast love	Ruth and Naomi
strengthened faith	the Widow at Zarephath and her son
hope	the Israelites
protection and/or security	
understanding	Daniel, Hananiah, Mishael and Azariah
help being faithful to God	Mephibosheth
a reunion	Prophets of the LORD
favor and honor	Jacob's family
news to share of God's goodness	the large crowd
restored life	
more insight into God's character	

Does God still help through people? Is it God's will for us to do anything?

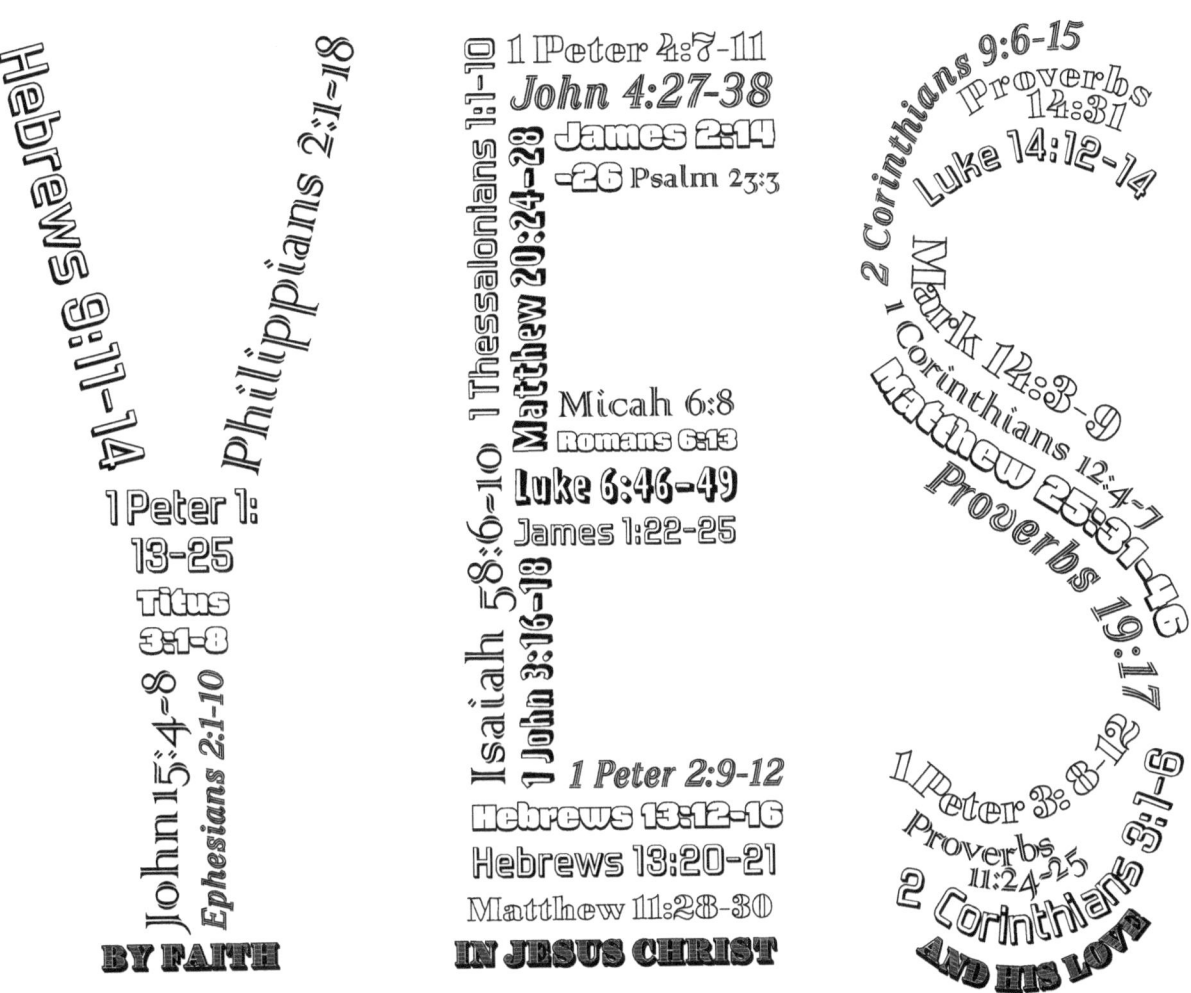

The "YES" is formed from Bible verse references:

Y (BY FAITH)
- Hebrews 9:11-14
- Philippians 2:1-18
- 1 Peter 1:13-25
- Titus 3:1-8
- John 15:4-8
- Ephesians 2:1-10

E (IN JESUS CHRIST)
- 1 Peter 4:7-11
- John 4:27-38
- James 2:14-26
- Psalm 23:3
- 1 Thessalonians 1:1-10
- Matthew 20:24-28
- Isaiah 58:6-10
- 1 John 3:16-18
- Micah 6:8
- Romans 6:13
- Luke 6:46-49
- James 1:22-25
- 1 Peter 2:9-12
- Hebrews 13:12-16
- Hebrews 13:20-21
- Matthew 11:28-30

S (AND HIS LOVE)
- 2 Corinthians 9:6-15
- Proverbs 14:31
- Luke 14:12-14
- 2 Corinthians 1
- Mark 12:3-9
- 1 Corinthians 12:4-7
- Matthew 25:31-46
- Proverbs 19:17
- 1 Peter 3:8-12
- Proverbs 11:24-25
- 2 Corinthians 3:1-6

At the start, we took a brief look at what volunteers do at food banks. While volunteering can be a way we put love in action, it's certainly not the only help we can give, it's not always what is needed, and it isn't something that we must do to serve God. While what we do may differ, it is clear that God intends for us to be doers of good. The 'YES' verses each shed a little light on the good God calls us to in Christ.

The verses on page 41 are not a checklist of things we must do to be saved. We cannot earn salvation; it's God's gift to us through Jesus Christ! Why should we care, then, what God has said beyond the message of forgiveness through the love, sacrifice and blood of Jesus Christ? Because our Savior, the risen Christ, is also our Lord whom we now love and are glad to follow, with the Word of God as the light to our path. Of course, we're not yet saved from the presence of sin, so we still struggle and fall short all too often, but God's grace is greater. What a relief that God made Himself our salvation! He will not lose any of His own.

Love is essential to our response of faith, being both why we listen to God and what God calls us to in Christ. As you read these verses, remember that God empowers and nurtures love in His people.

1 John 4:7~21	John 14:15~17	John 15:1~17	Galatians 5:1~26	1 Corinthians 13
Philippians 2:1~8	Colossians 3:12~17	Luke 6:27~36	Romans 12:9~21	Romans 13:8~14
2 Timothy 3:1~9	2 Peter 1:1~9	1 John 2:15~17	1 John 3:11~18	& 1 John 5:1~5

Read Ephesians 5:1~2. Starting at "Love" in the top left, highlight the path that describes love God's way. Except for the first and last, each hexagon borders with two in the path: the previous one and the next one.

Love — begins with God's love for us — is not given to enemies — is kind — protects — is faithful — trusts — comforts — lives in fearful dread — gives what's deserved always — is easy — is merciful — can be hard and cost us here — helps unless it gets too heavy — exalts Christ, crucified & risen

begins with duty — serves self — leaves to fend for self — doubts — flares up and dies — obeys what is good — uses helping for own status — honors others above self

serves others — is patient — is envious — stays in hope — is never tempted — goes its own way — is generous

must be sincere — holds grudges — rejoices with/for others — has a limited supply — doesn't give evil for evil — doesn't give evil for evil — helps whoever gives back — is only feelings

is prideful — seeks revenge — honors the truth — bears with one another — is overcome by desire — cares and takes action — is often a choice

is humble — leads us to repent — delights in evil — honors all ways — overcomes — is by human power — comes from God's Spirit

is slow to anger — honors forgiveness from God — makes our joy full

is never angry — turns a blind eye to sin — pursues peace — doesn't speak up ever — is mature(d)

This activity does not go over everything about love, but it does give us practice recognizing God's way of love. Whether or not you needed help to know the path, each of us need God's forgiveness and help daily to live it.

We don't naturally have the love God calls us to be abounding in, but, thankfully, this love is grown by God in all who live by faith in Jesus Christ. How? Do you remember the crossword activity? Through the verses shared there, we learned a lot about how God gives and develops His righteousness in us, like how He gives us the Spirit of Christ who transforms us through His Word. God also grows us through and for His Church.

Write each word in its matching empty piece. The first is already filled. Read from the top, left to right.

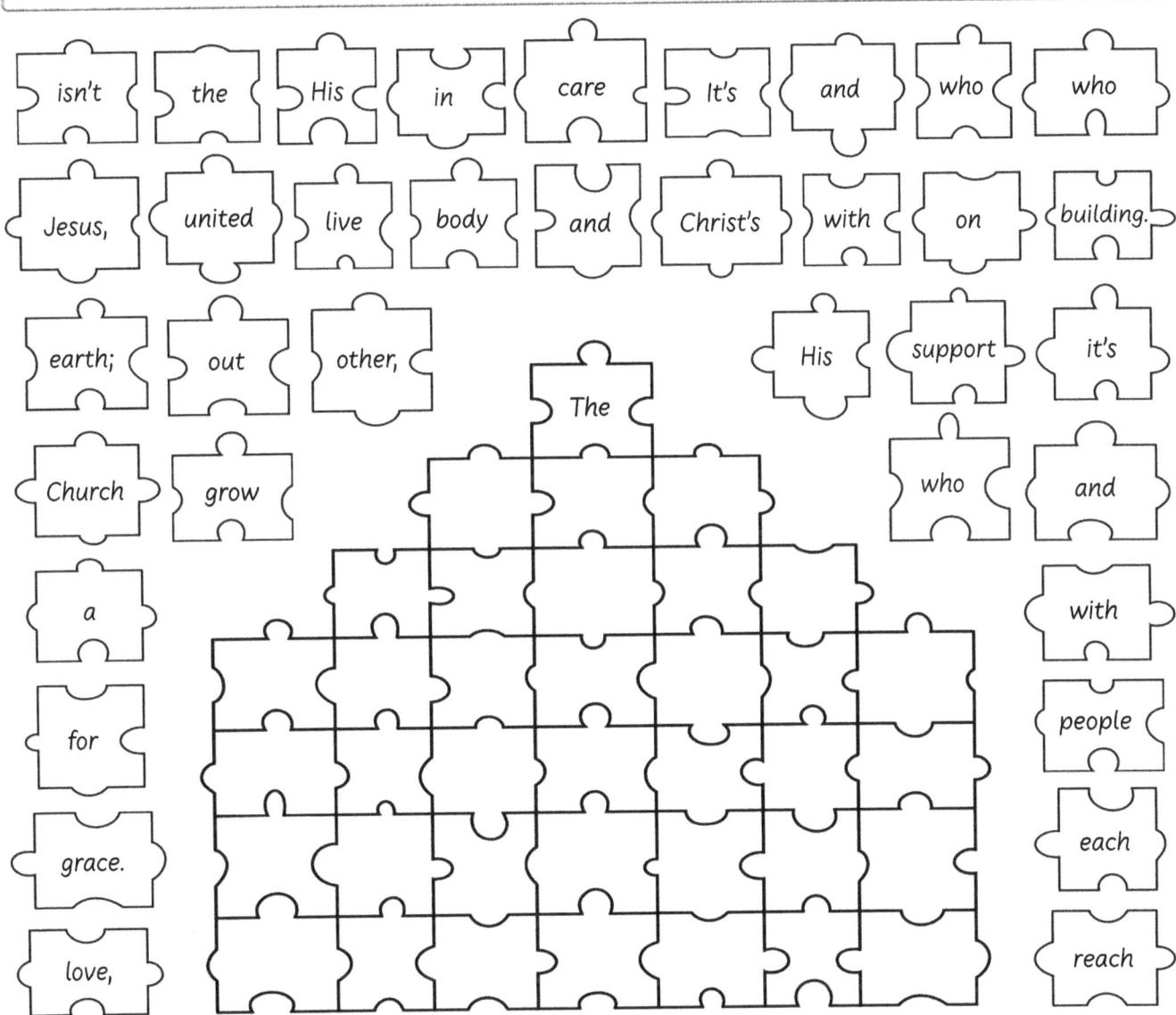

isn't · the · His · in · care · It's · and · who · who

Jesus, · united · live · body · and · Christ's · with · on · building.

earth; · out · other, · The · His · support · it's

Church · grow · who · and

a · with

for · people

grace. · each

love, · reach

A jigsaw puzzle is not a perfect picture of the Church, but it does help bring some things into focus.

A jigsaw puzzle shows us the importance of each piece, each person, being found. See Luke 15:1~7!

It shows how, sometimes, when one piece (one person!) is added, that leads to others around it also being found and brought into the same state of security that the one just entered. See John 4:1~42.

It shows with every piece how the Church and Kingdom of God grows closer to completion as more and more are found, reconciled, and unified with Christ and with His people. See Ephesians 2:1~22.

It shows by its very design the intent for and blessing of community and fellowship. See 1 John 1:3~7.

In the same way, it shows that Church members are meant to give real support to and receive it from one another. See 2 Corinthians 1:3~11, Galatians 6:7~10, Hebrews 3:12~14, and 1 Peter 4:8~11.

It shows the uniqueness we have been made and gifted with and how the Church, as Christ's body, needs each one for wholeness in being and function. See Romans 12:3~8 and 1 Corinthians 12:4~20.

It shows unity in how, even though puzzles are built in various sections (like local churches), they are all part of the same puzzle (the Church) and will be brought together one day. See Ephesians 4:1~6.

And a puzzle, as a representation of the Church, glorifies God because what puzzle piece could be found and secured without a greater being? For a puzzle, of course, that's simply us people. For the Church, that's amazingly God the Father through Jesus Christ and His Holy Spirit. See 1 Peter 1:1~5.

Unlike puzzles, which are not able to bring in its pieces, we are called to help build the Kingdom—not because we ourselves are able, but because God has given us His Holy Spirit as well as gifts to use for His Kingdom, because God Himself is reaching out and working through us. See 2 Corinthians 3:1~6.

Unlike puzzles which only grow in size as pieces are filled in, Church members also grow and mature personally in Christ, like in the ways we learned about during the crossword. See Ephesians 4:11~16.

Unlike puzzle pieces, we go home from group gatherings of Church members and we remain in the world for our daily lives. Still, whether we are together or apart, we belong to our Savior and we live to honor Him—He is our worthy Lord always, not just on Sunday mornings! See John 17:1~2, 13~26.

Unlike puzzles and their pieces, which have no relationship with the people who enjoy them, we are so loved by God, and filled by God, and made for joyful life forever with God. See Ephesians 3:14~21!

One does not have to be a believer and follower of Jesus Christ to serve people, but His true Church has the unique reality, significance, and responsibility of being the body of Christ here, sent into the world with hope from the Holy Spirit; with compassion and help; with the Bread of Life and the Word of God.

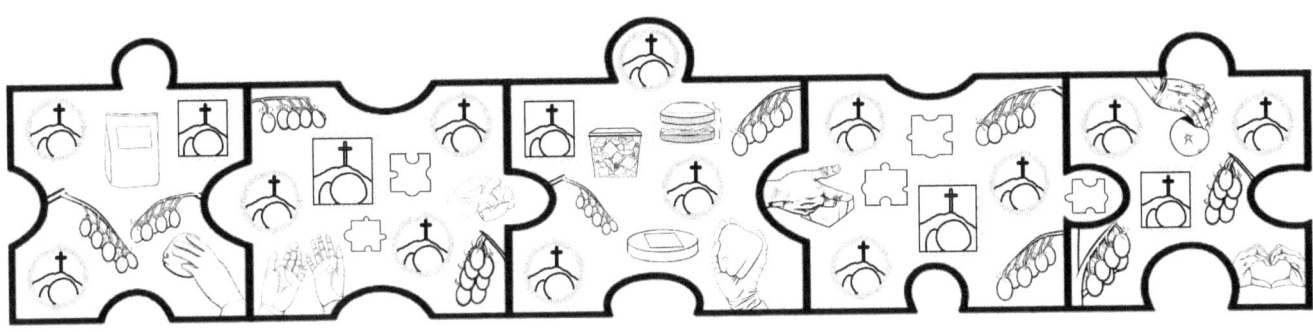

How many symbols/pictures are in each of the above puzzle pieces? __ __ __ __ __
Adding all of those numbers together = _____. Multiplying those same numbers instead = _____.

Individual faithfulness is significant in its impact because it is God's Holy Spirit working in and through us. How much more might God do through us when we are encouraging one another in doing God's good will (see Hebrews 10:19-25) and are responding in faith together? This increase is more like multiplying than adding and is far better than we could imagine or do in our own power! Remember Ephesians 3:20-21?!

This is really awesome! But we may start to wonder something that needs to be addressed so that we do not become burdened beyond God's will. As the body of Christ, through the Spirit of God in us,

CAN THE CHURCH END HUNGER?

Fully and finally for all who live? No. This is promised to be done through Jesus Christ after His return. Does that mean we are to do nothing or that anything we do to help fight hunger is actually in vain? No! Remember, we've been reading that God can, wants to, and does make real differences in people's lives through people. And His Church not only has helping hands to give, but the heart of Christ and the message of our living hope, the same one that brought us to Jesus—to life, faith and peace in Him. And even when their/our situations are not changing, God is always, always working all things for the good of His people. So, may we, the Church, put faith and love in action as God calls us to, in the name and grace of our Lord Jesus Christ, shining His light and giving His help in this dark and difficult world by the Holy Spirit's guidance and power until God brings every word and promise of His to fulfillment.

For all who are experiencing or witnessing suffering, I hope this gives you comfort and encouragement.

Really struggling with suffering does not mean we have no faith. What matters is how we respond. Do we let it be something that turns us away from God, or do we go to God and to His Word for help? Since we are not taken out of the world right when we first believe, there are many hard and terrible things we must face with faith. When we do not understand something in our life or in the world, the truth that we do know from and about God is always enough to keep trusting Him wholeheartedly.

Let's practice turning to truths that are helpful to remember whenever we're struggling spiritually because of suffering. With each statement, think of a Bible passage (shared in this book or from your own reading) that reminds you that this is true and trustworthy no matter what. Write them here.

We know God is good, wise, and all-powerful; that He cares, takes action, and always keeps His Word.

We know that Jesus understands our suffering and promises His people mercy, healing, and justice.

We know that God works even the bad things we face here for our good and that death is not the end.

Also, read Luke 16:19-31. This parable from Jesus does not mean that all people who are poor will be in heaven, but it does show God's heart for the poor and warns us about not listening to His Word.

Along with repeating the encouragement to turn to God's unchanging Word, below are helpful things to put into practice always and especially when you're struggling in any way. Keep in mind that these suggestions are not a formula for getting God's help in the way or timing we want, but, rather, are real ways we may exercise the faith that God's given us and be helped by God in our mind, heart, and spirit even while we're still in the midst of our trails, needing to wait on God and trust Him with everything.

These are surely easier said than done. We need the compassionate help of God to follow through even on these small but significant acts of faith, especially in hard, overwhelming, and devastating times. Let's go to Him.

Seek God's Word to remember His character, His promises, and His deeds. Ask God to strengthen your faith in Him. Perhaps start with Psalm 103, Hebrews 1:1~4, Matthew 6:25~33, and Romans 8:28~39.

Think through and thank God for the ways He has been providing for you. Ask God to open your eyes when you need help seeing His presence in your life. He is always with His own (see Matthew 28:20).

Pour out your heart to God in prayer (see Psalm 62). God knows it all, of course, but He wants you to take all your worries and needs to Him. He promises to fill you with His peace (see Philippians 4:4~9). He loves you and wants you to always cast your cares on Him (see 1 Peter 5:6~11). Through Christ, God has given us the ability and the confidence to go right to Him in prayer (see Hebrews 4:14~16).

Wait. God hears and answers in His good way the prayers of the humble—seeking or saved by Christ. See Psalm 66:16~20 and 145:18~19, Isaiah 66:2, Romans 8:23~26, 1 Peter 3:12, and 1 John 5:13~15.

Don't let doubts take hold. Fellow believers are going through similar things (see 1 Peter 5:8~9 again). Stay honest with your family and friends in the Church. God's comfort is often given through them (see 2 Corinthians 1:1~7). Likewise, keep your heart open to anyone God might comfort through you.

Let your heart rest, knowing whose hands you are in. See John 10:27~30, Psalm 23, and Luke 12:32.

Rejoice in the victory of our Lord Jesus Christ and in how God mercifully and graciously makes us heirs of the Kingdom through Him. Whatever troubles and severe trials we might go through here are not nothing—they matter deeply to God—but, in view of eternity with God, they really cannot compare with the absolute glory that is to come (see Romans 8:14~25 and 2 Corinthians 4:16~18). Hallelujah!!

Read the Parable of the Four Soils in Mark 4:1~20.

If we have truly become rooted in Jesus Christ by faith, no suffering, even from our spiritual enemy, will cause us to lose our faith and salvation because our Savior is the source of our life and eternal security. The same is true for when weeds threaten our faith, but it is good to remember that living by faith in God means we listen to His Word—in this case, as He warns of the weeds that choke out faith. What weeds should we watch for? Jesus explains them to be worry, the deceitfulness of wealth, and worldly desires.

Use the key to fill in the letters.

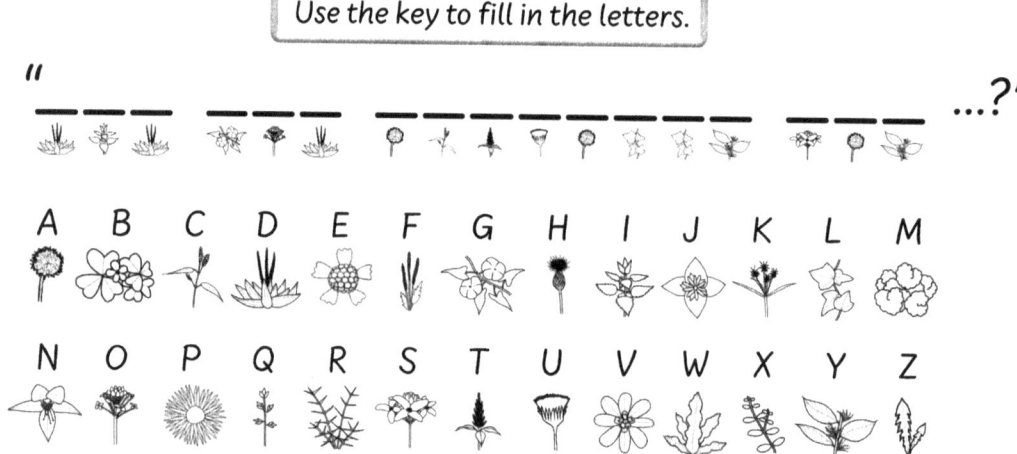

Remember Genesis 3? That's still a way the devil preys on people, coming for us by any means possible to challenge God and His Word. How does this method make it easier for weeds to rapidly overwhelm us?

Let's look briefly at each weed. Worry can shoot up in anyone, especially in times of hardship and need. Deeply rooted worry can cause a hard battle as the devil preys on us, but victory isn't won by us, it's won by the Bread of Life; the Light of the World that darkness will never overcome; the Door of the Sheep, our Good Shepherd; the Resurrection and the Life; the Way, the Truth, and the Life; the True Vine. Remember His faithfulness and love, His care for every detail of our lives, His total authority and readiness to help us. Go back to page 47 for the encouragements and verses there and definitely go to God. His peace prevails.

As to wealth, it is not that having money or things is wrong in itself, but we must take seriously all that God has said, commanded, and warned about them and their place in our hearts, such as Psalm 37:16, Matthew 6:19-24 & 16:26, Luke 12:13-34, 2 Corinthians 9:6-15, 1 Timothy 6:3-19, & Hebrews 13:5-16.

Read James 2:14-17. How might you respond in faith when you know of someone's need for food? I am sure you can give some great answers to that question already. Read Luke 3:11 as well. Simple? But, look... around this plant of faith in Christ are possible weeds that could keep faith from being fruitful in love, kindness, goodness, gentleness, and faithfulness, as shown through compassion. For all who believe, and, thus, who listen to God, what truths might God's Spirit bring to mind and to bear in our lives to uproot and overcome these weeds?

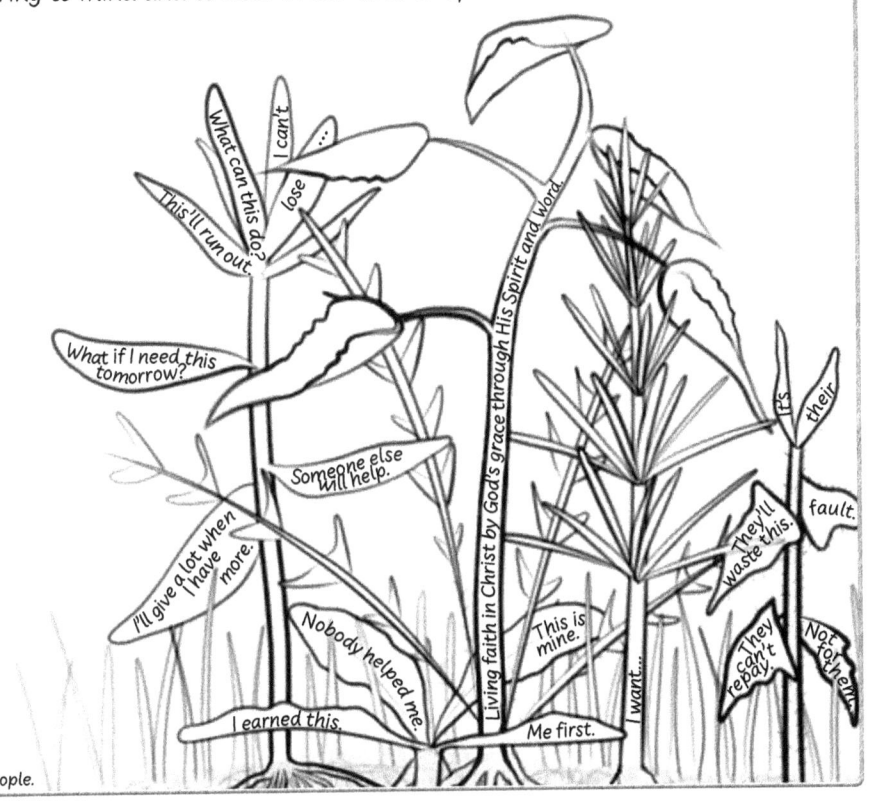

Note: this is not me telling you to always give money to people.

As to worldly desires, it is not that God does not want us to enjoy life, for He surely does, but, once we've been brought to life in Christ, we no longer live for the moment in pursuit of or being pleased by the very ways from which Jesus redeemed us. Even with our hearts fixed on Jesus and His eternal Kingdom, these desires are tempting with shows, ads, social media and more telling us what the 'good life' is, but we're not on our own. Our God knows how to develop and truly satisfy our hunger and thirst for righteousness. Read Romans 6:1-14 and Galatians 5:16-24 again, as well as Ephesians 4:17-24 and 1 Peter 2:11-12.

With a message that urges us to love actively, it's important we hear what Jesus says in Matthew 6:1~4. Please read it.

Can you think of any modern-day things that we wield like trumpets to announce our "good" deeds?

God warns us many times to watch out for and not follow people who are only outwardly religious, who are not truly united by faith to Jesus Christ, who are motivated by status, pride, and personal benefits.

Does this mean we have to be secret followers of Jesus, only worshiping, obeying, and serving God when we are alone and are sure that only God will know? No. Remember 1 Peter 2:11~12? There, the Holy Spirit says through Peter that people may see the reality of our faith in Jesus, to the glory of God. Likewise, read what Jesus says in Matthew 5:13~16. It is okay to be seen living by faith in God; people will naturally see since true faith is not turned on and off. Believers in Jesus are called and empowered by God to do good (remember Ephesians 2:10, Galatians 6:10, and Titus 3:8?), but we must be watchful and not turn back to following the world's way, which is marked by faith in oneself, pride in oneself, and service for oneself.

Read 1 Corinthians 13:1~3. Why are all these things that seem so good to people actually nothing to God?

What did Jesus say about the Vine and our fruitfulness or lack of fruit in John 15 (especially in verse 5)?

God cultivates humility in us not to make us feel bad about ourselves, but to keep us genuinely and gladly dependent on the only one who is truly able to give, grow, and sustain real righteousness in us—Himself. Read Psalm 130 and Philippians 1:9~11!

As God's redeemed people, His children adopted through Jesus Christ, what is good fuel for our motives?

It is important we keep remembering that we do not obey in order to become God's children; rather, good becomes what we want to do and are led and helped to do because we are, because our hearts, changed and filled with God's Holy Spirit, are being grown by our good Father in unity with His own heart. Amen!

With words or drawings, fill in the pieces with different ways that we might reflect the heart of God. You can also add specific ways we could put the two that have already been written into practice.

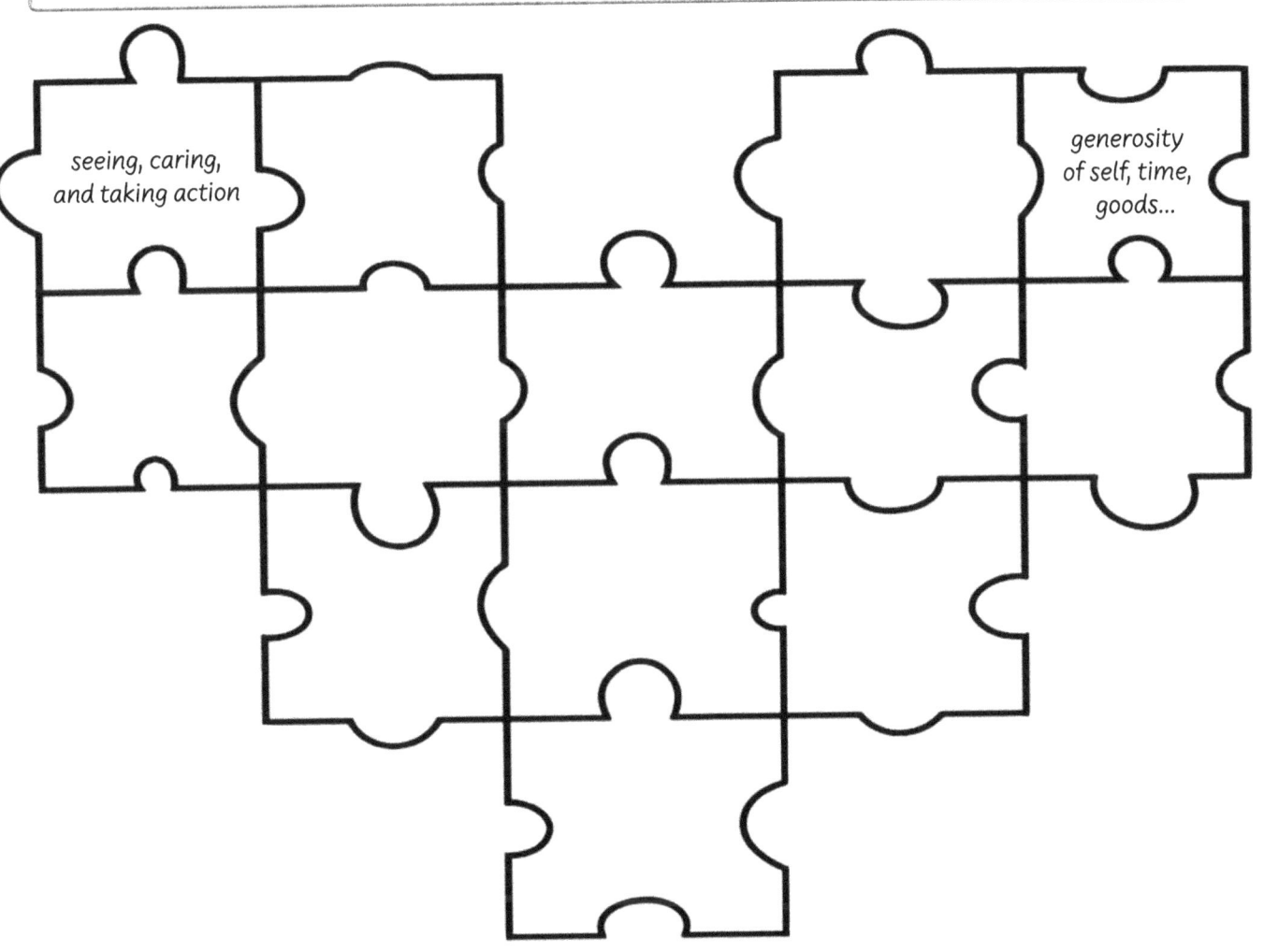

seeing, caring, and taking action

generosity of self, time, goods...

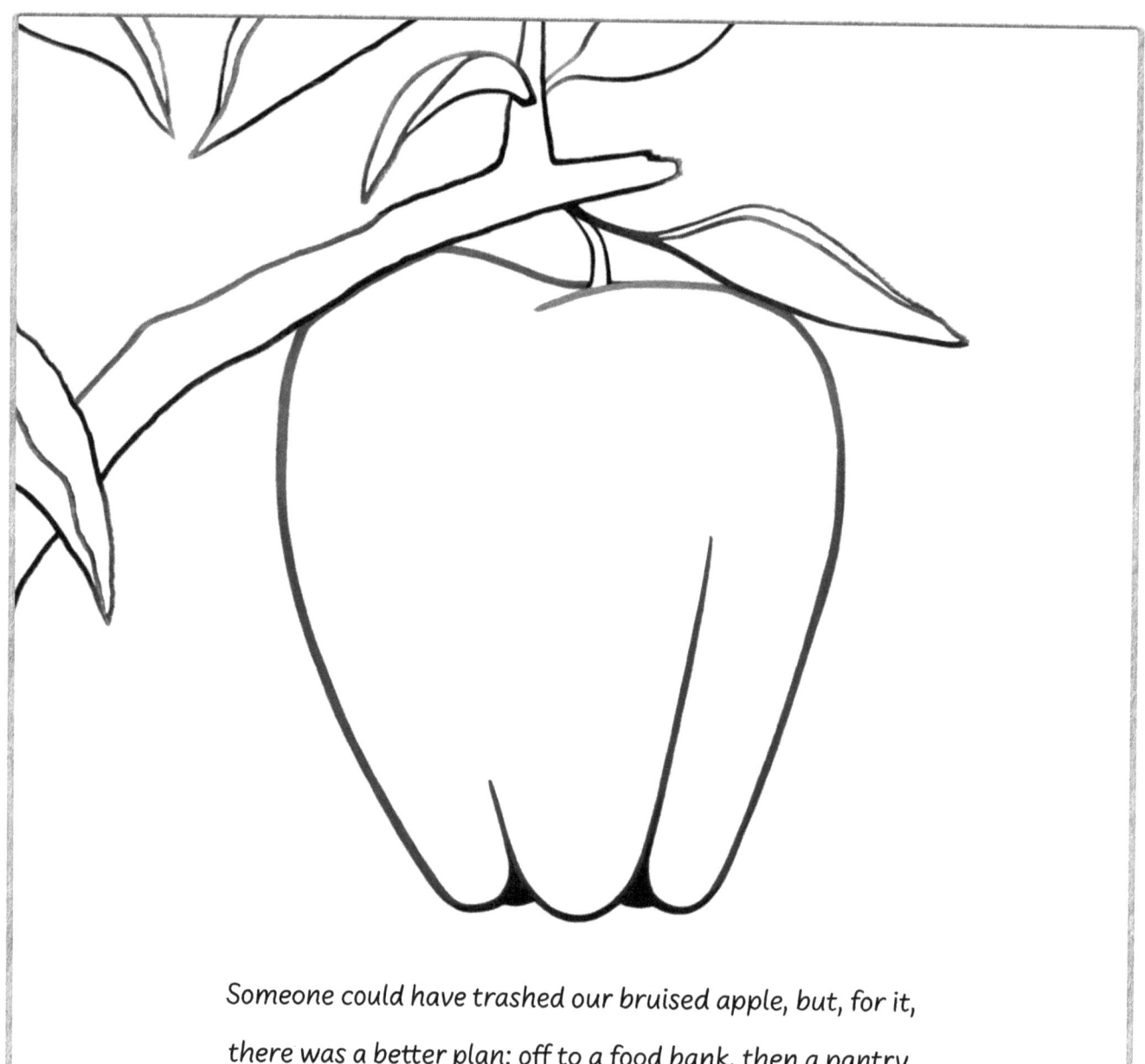

Someone could have trashed our bruised apple, but, for it,

there was a better plan: off to a food bank, then a pantry,

and into the hands of a young man.

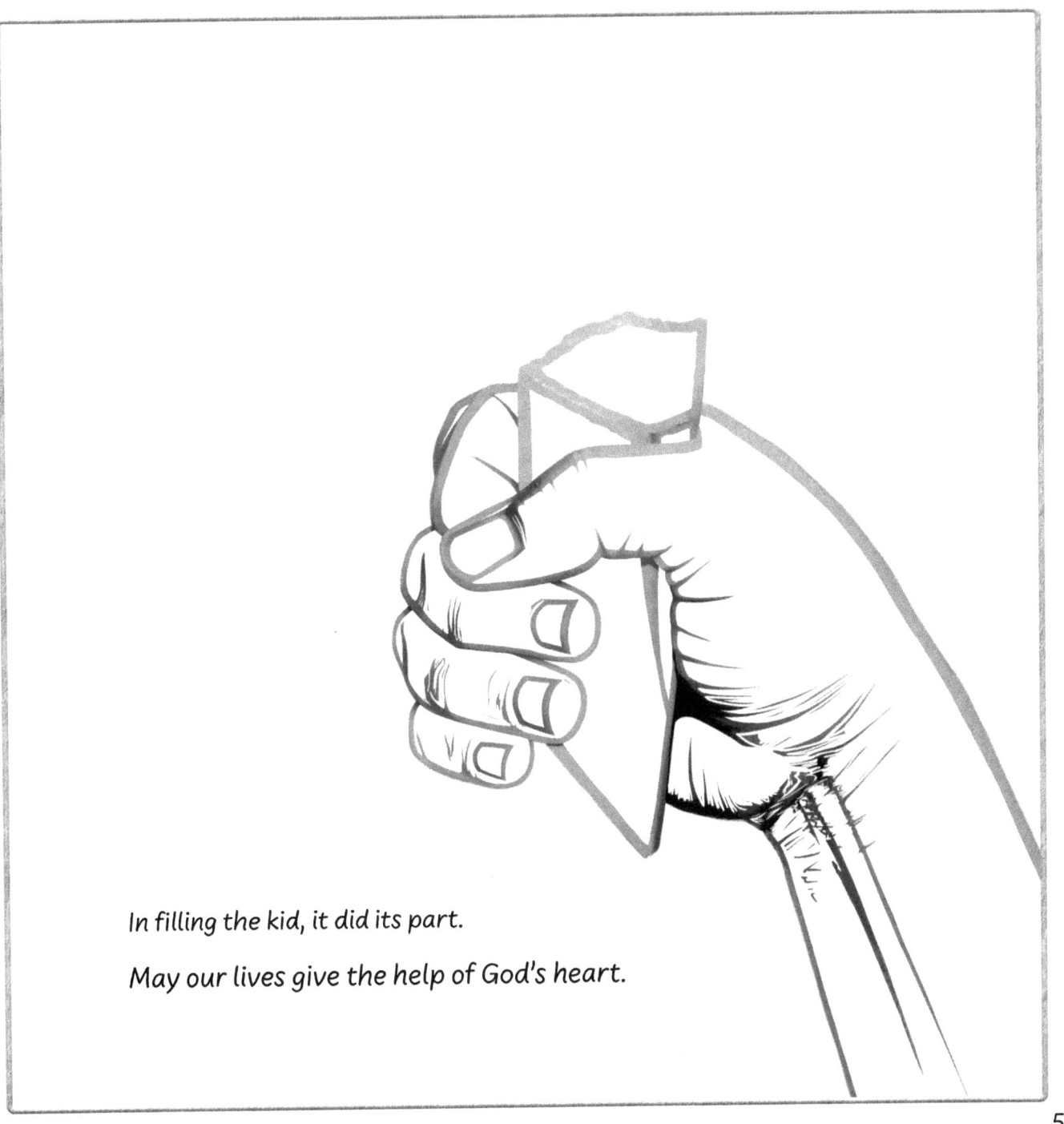

In filling the kid, it did its part.

May our lives give the help of God's heart.

Summary (un)Scramble!

For help or after unscrambling, look up the verse listed beside it. To be sure that word is in the translation, use the ESV (English Standard Version) or the NIV (New International Version).

Psalm 34:8	aestt	_ _ _ _ _
Ephesians 1:7	ridpneteom	_ _ _ _ _ _ _ _ _ _
1 Peter 1:3	iigvnl	_ _ _ _ _ _
Psalm 146:5	pheo	_ _ _ _
Romans 8:17	rcdnihle	_ _ _ _ _ _ _ _
Philippians 4:11	tonncte	_ _ _ _ _ _ _
Psalm 37:16	tlleit	_ _ _ _ _ _
Psalm 145:19	slfliufl	_ _ _ _ _ _ _ _
Psalm 23:5	beatl	_ _ _ _ _
1 Peter 5:6	mhlbue	_ _ _ _ _ _
Philippians 4:7	paeec	_ _ _ _ _
John 15:5	ncbehrsa	_ _ _ _ _ _ _ _
Hebrews 9:14	freedfo	_ _ _ _ _ _ _
Matthew 5:6	lsbseed	_ _ _ _ _ _ _
Philippians 1:11	lyorg	_ _ _ _ _
2 Peter 1:3	vienid	_ _ _ _ _ _
2 Corinthians 1:4	ormctfo	_ _ _ _ _ _ _
1 Peter 4:10	resev	_ _ _ _ _
Galatians 6:10	odgo	_ _ _ _
Psalm 62:8	ufegre	_ _ _ _ _ _
Hebrews 4:16	eecrvie	_ _ _ _ _ _ _
Romans 8:37	nroqecsoru	_ _ _ _ _ _ _ _ _ _
2 Peter 3:13	oseirpm	_ _ _ _ _ _ _
Matthew 25:34	parpeder	_ _ _ _ _ _ _ _

because of

Iniquity
Human weakness to think, say, and do wrong. The reason we will not and also cannot save ourselves.

Justice
Everyone held fully accountable with no excuses, loopholes or bribes to get off—only fair judgments.

Wrath
God's rightful judgment for sin. What Jesus, in our stead, took entirely; what unbelievers will receive.

Confess
Admit our sins (especially to God), having sincere sorrow and desiring to be forgiven and reconciled.

Reconciled
In a relationship of peace, restored by forgiveness and characterized by enjoyment of righteousness.

Righteous / Righteousness
Believing in Christ, Jesus' record counted as ours. / The fruition of Christ's work and Spirit within us.

Grace
Undeserved and abundant blessing / favor / good, freely given entirely from the good will of the giver.

Merciful
Ready, able, & desiring to pardon the contrite, not giving what's deserved to gladly give compassion.

Salvation
Rescue from self, sin, evil, death, & deserved wrath into God's love, peace, righteousness, & eternal life.

Repentance
Turning from sin and our ways to God and His way by the grace of God in Christ (see Acts 11:14-18).

Faith [in God]
Trust in God; confidence in God's Word, character, promises, and victorious power (see Hebrews 11).

Good Works [e.g. Ephesians 2:10]
What believers do following Jesus by God's Spirit, with hope in and from God, not in or from ourself.

His great Love ~ Ephesians 2:4

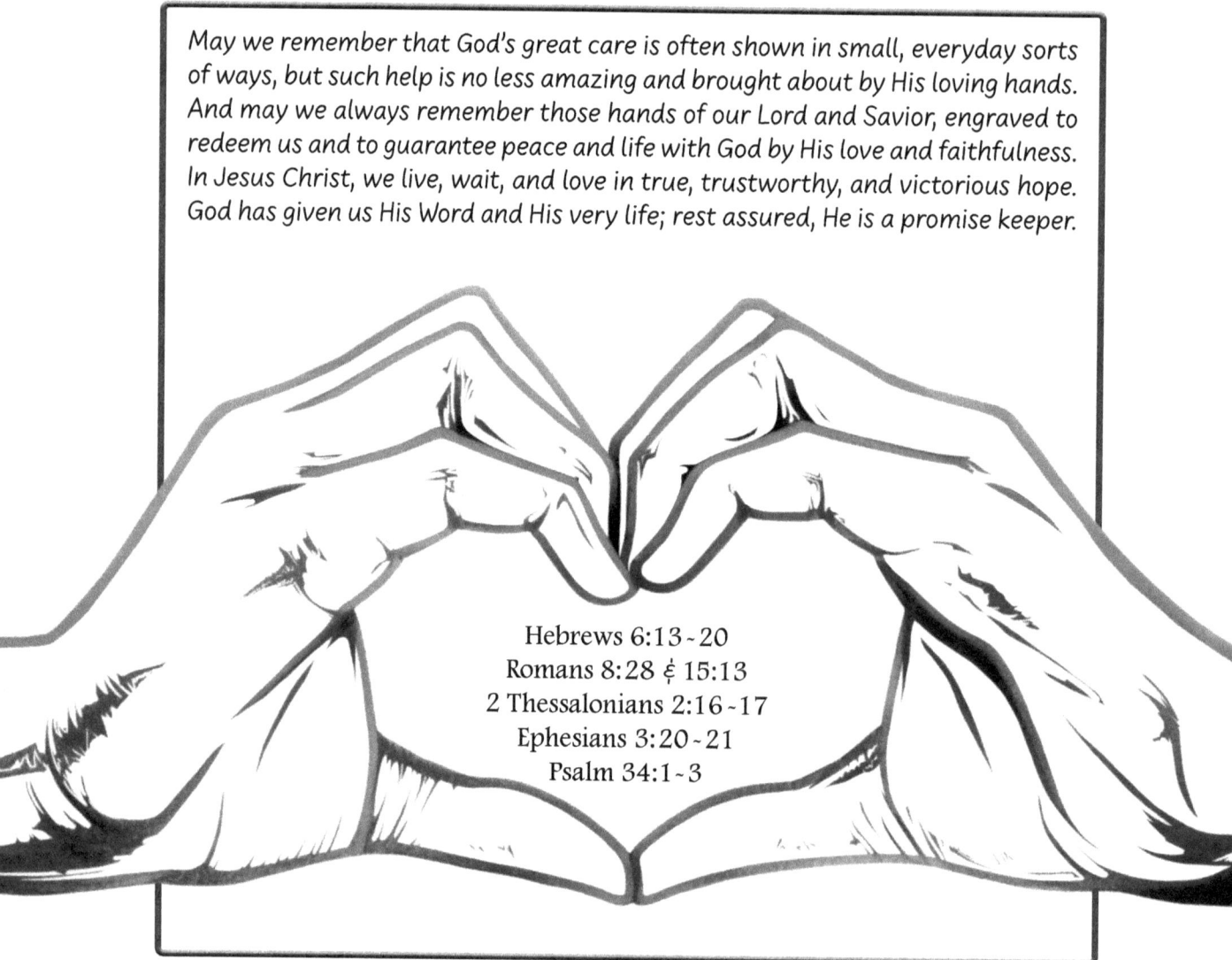

May we remember that God's great care is often shown in small, everyday sorts of ways, but such help is no less amazing and brought about by His loving hands. And may we always remember those hands of our Lord and Savior, engraved to redeem us and to guarantee peace and life with God by His love and faithfulness. In Jesus Christ, we live, wait, and love in true, trustworthy, and victorious hope. God has given us His Word and His very life; rest assured, He is a promise keeper.

Hebrews 6:13~20
Romans 8:28 & 15:13
2 Thessalonians 2:16~17
Ephesians 3:20~21
Psalm 34:1~3

www.ingramcontent.com/pod-product-compliance
Lightning Source LLC
Chambersburg PA
CBHW041541120626
46551CB00019B/2797